<u>You</u> Can Control Diabetes

A personal guide to self-empowerment

By Abdul Ghani, MD
and
Gary Scheiner, MS, CDE

Published by:
Midtown Publishing Company

Disclaimer
The examples and explanations given in this book are presented for educational purposes only and may not apply to your individual situation. The reader is reminded to always consult his/her personal physician concerning changes in medical therapy.

TABLE OF CONTENTS

Acknowledgments

Dr. Ghani

I want to thank my teachers, S. K. Bhatia, MD and Gerald Burke, MD who taught me so much about diabetes when I was at Cook County Hospital in Chicago in the mid-1970s. I want to thank Karen Colovin, Margo Smith and Blake McDonald for helping to prepare the manuscript. I want to thank my patients who have taught me so much. I want to thank my family and friends for their moral support, especially Fauzia Ghani, Sarah Ghani, Howard M. Cloke III, and Pamela Zipperer-Davis.

Gary Scheiner

My sincerest appreciation to my wife Deborah who changed most of our daughter Marley's diapers while I was busy writing, and encouraged me to "go for it." Thank you to my parents, Sara and Paul Scheiner, for giving me the confidence and inspiration to manage my own diabetes and share my ideas with others. Special thanks to the people at the Juvenile Diabetes Foundation, American Diabetes Association, American Association of Diabetes Educators and International Diabetic Athletes Association for their ongoing commitment to teaching and assisting people with diabetes.

We would also like to thank the following people for reviewing the book:

Lois Babione, RN, RD, CDE; Pius Jacob, MD; Orlando J. Castillo, MD; Liaquat Allarakhia, MD; David M. Klachko, MD; Marvin E. Levin, MD; David S. Schade, MD; and Mark Burge, MD.

Preface

There must be at least 20 different books out there on diabetes management. What in the world would possess someone to read (or write) another?

First of all, diabetes is a chronic disease that affects more than 16 million Americans. That's a lot of people! And the number is going to keep growing as our population ages and becomes more overweight. People with poorly controlled diabetes are suffering from blindness, kidney failure, loss of limbs, heart disease and major nerve disorders that wind up costing our country more than 110 *billion* dollars annually (that's one out of every six dollars spent on health care!).

Next, more than 90% of people with diabetes do not see specialists; they are treated by family doctors (primary care physicians) who, in most cases, received only *two days* of training on diabetes in medical school. In this age of specialized, assembly-line health care, most doctors do not have the time or skills necessary to manage a challenging disease like diabetes.

The assumption that health care providers have made until now is that people with diabetes are not capable of managing themselves. The health care industry has kept some of the most important concepts (such as medication dosage adjustment and dietary flexibility) out of the hands of the patients who can use and benefit from them. As a result, millions of people are suffering and dying because they did not get the information and training they needed.

The purpose of this book is to teach you how to do a better job of managing your own diabetes, safely.

Diabetes is a disease of *lifestyle*. It forces us to make countless decisions that will affect control on a day-to-day basis. Nevertheless, people continue to rely heavily on their physicians for direction in all facets of their health, even when it comes to basic day-to-day issues and decision-making. As managed care becomes a dominant force in the health care system, patients cannot continue to rely on the physician to do all the decision making for them.

The time is now to take diabetes care out of the waiting room and put it where it belongs - into the living room.

The time is right to start taking control of your own diabetes. With new medications, insulin delivery devices, food choices, blood sugar monitoring systems and the ability to make safe, intelligent adjustments to insulin and medication, just about anyone can improve their blood sugar control. And with new screening procedures and treatment options, complications of diabetes can be caught early and corrected before they lead to serious problems.

Becoming skilled at diabetes self-management does not mean that your physician no longer plays an important role. It simply means that your doctor is more of an expert adviser than a dictator of "do's" and "don'ts".

In this book you will be empowered to regulate your blood glucose levels, adjust insulin and oral medications (when, how and why), understand and manage the factors that raise and lower blood sugar levels (food, stress, exercise, etc.), seek out medical examinations and laboratory tests when needed, and basically do what it takes to successfully manage diabetes and prevent its complications.

Unlike other books on the same subject, this one is not afraid to share medical secrets and tell you exactly what needs to be done. It is not written for doctors, but for the average person who is trying to live a full and fulfilling life with diabetes. The information contained here is also up-to-date, including the latest diabetes medications, therapies, and methods of treatment.

The time is now to get started, and get in better control. You can do it!

Abdul Ghani, MD
Gary Scheiner, MS, CDE

FOREWORD

For nearly one hundred years, diabetes research has been one of the finest success stories of modern medicine. To people with diabetes, however, it must seem like the pace of research is plodding and that science has provided few tangible benefits. In fact, diabetes treatment has remained largely unchanged since the discovery of insulin in 1921. But this predicament is finally changing. Over the past several years, questions that have been debated for decades have been settled. For example, we now know that intensive management of diabetes with near-normalization of blood sugars will prevent many of the dreaded complications of the disease. As a result, diabetes treatment is changing. New diabetes medications have become available that are safer and more effective than ever before, and new strategies are available to help people with diabetes achieve the goal of "near normal blood sugar." The end result is more flexible and effective treatment for people with diabetes.

These advances could not have come at a better time. As the population of the United States ages, the number of people with diabetes is growing rapidly. There are currently 16 million people with diabetes in America, and although 40% of people over the age of 65 either have diabetes or pre-diabetes, only a fraction of these people have had their condition diagnosed and are thus able to begin treatment. The question of how to care for all of these people in a cost-effective manner is a critical issue for the medical profession over the coming decades. Experts agree that the best solution to this problem is for people with diabetes to assume much of the responsibility for caring for themselves and staying healthy. To accomplish this, however, requires a high level of understanding on the part of people with diabetes.

Dr. Ghani's and Mr. Scheiner's book, _You Can Control Diabetes_, is an important tool that can be used by people with diabetes to take charge of their condition and optimize their health. By presenting all of the fundamentals of diabetes care, as well as news about the latest advances in diabetes research, in an entertaining and understandable manner, Dr. Ghani and Mr. Scheiner provide people with diabetes the information they need to achieve the goal of safe, effective, and affordable diabetes care. I recommend that people read the book from cover to cover, and then save the book as a reference resource. Family members may also benefit from reading the book. Those with diabetes will probably benefit most from a stepwise approach to improving their diabetes care. This means choosing one aspect of diabetes care to improve and incorporating these changes into your daily routine. Once this task has been mastered and has become "easy", then you can begin to incorporate a new task. This book is full of suggestions, stories, strategies and solutions that can help anyone with diabetes improve their health.

So good luck as you continue your journey with diabetes. Remember to appreciate the challenge and to take pride in your accomplishments. Every small step in improving your diabetes control is a step towards a longer, healthier life.

Mark R. Burge, MD
Assistant Professor of Medicine
Endocrinology and Metabolism
University of New Mexico Health Sciences Center
Albuquerque, NM

Section I

Diabetes – What is it? What does it do? And why the heck did I get it?

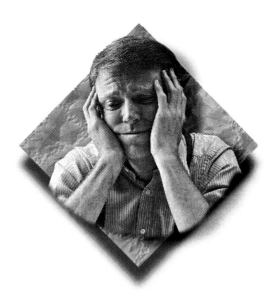

Chapter 1: What is diabetes?

A few months ago, a young woman walked into my office looking like she just pulled an all-nighter. She was tired, thirsty, and had the same glazed-over look that many of us get when our spouses start talking about china patterns. She had lost a lot of weight over the past couple of months, and was running to the bathroom every 15 minutes.

When the lab tests came back and she was told she had diabetes, her only comment was, "Are you sure we have to treat it? I never lost weight this easily in my life!"

Diabetes can be a dangerous and deadly illness if you let it have its way with you. Many people have years taken off their lives by diabetes. And many spend the latter part of their lives suffering the pain and frustration that comes with diabetic complications. What's most frustrating is that most of this suffering could be avoided if people would take better care of themselves. Take care of your diabetes, and chances are very good that you will lead a full and healthy life. Rather than lying in a hospital bed with tubes sticking out of you, you'll be able to travel the world and dance at your granddaughter's wedding.

Diabetes management is like a big, beautiful home with lots of floors and intricate fixtures. But in order to keep the house standing, you have to have a solid foundation. Your basic understanding of diabetes is the foundation that we will build upon throughout this book.

The role of insulin...

Diabetes is a condition in which the body is unable to convert the food we eat into energy. When a person without diabetes eats food, most of the food is broken down into a simple sugar called glucose. The glucose is carried in the bloodstream to all the cells of the body where it is burned for energy.

Insulin is a substance produced by the pancreas (an organ located just below the stomach) when we eat food. Any time the blood sugar rises, it "tickles" the pancreas to make more insulin. Insulin is required to get the sugar out of the bloodstream and into the body's cells (such as muscle cells and fat cells) so that it can be burned for energy. As a result, the blood sugar rarely rises above a certain level, 120 milligrams per deciliter (we'll just call it "120").

Besides helping get sugar out of the bloodstream and into the body's cells, Insulin has another job: storing sugar in the liver. Insulin is the "packer" that puts sugar into the liver for use at another time.

When a person has not eaten for a while, the blood sugar level can come down. This can occur between meals, during sleep, and especially during exercise. When the blood sugar level drops, the pancreas slows down its production of insulin. Not only does this reduce the amount of sugar being put into the body's cells, it also allows the liver to release some of the sugar that was stored up earlier. As a result, blood sugar levels don't go too low, rarely falling below "60".

In a way, the pancreas acts like the thermostat that keeps your house comfy cozy. When the temperature goes up, the thermostat kicks on the fan. When the temperature goes down, the thermostat kicks on the heat. That way, the temperature stays within a comfortable range of, say, 70 to 80 degrees.

In your body, when the blood sugar level begins to rise, the pancreas spits out insulin which brings the blood sugar level down. When the blood sugar level falls, the pancreas stops producing insulin and the blood sugar comes back up. This system helps keep the blood sugar within a range that is comfy-cozy for your body: 70 to 120.

Here Comes Trouble...

What if your thermostat broke in the middle of summer? The temperature would keep going up, and the fan wouldn't go on. Even if you turn the fan on manually, it might be too late to cool the house down.

Diabetes means that the blood sugar levels are too high because, quite simply, the insulin system is broken. If the pancreas stops producing insulin all together, we call it "Type-I" or "insulin-dependent" diabetes. It is usually caused by an autoimmune process in which our body's defense system attacks and slowly destroys the pancreas. A person with Type-I diabetes depends on insulin injections for basic survival.

The symptoms come on suddenly and can be quite severe. Very high blood sugar levels cause a person to urinate a great deal as the kidneys try to get rid of the sugar through the urine. In essence, you will be urinating away almost everything you eat. All the urinating can make you very thirsty. And since you will be unable to get sugar into your cells, your energy level will be low, and you will have to resort to fat as your only source of energy. Consequently, rapid weight loss can occur.

Without insulin injections, a person with Type-I diabetes will eventually go into a coma and die. Management of Type-I diabetes involves careful balancing of insulin, exercise and food so that blood sugar levels stay as close to normal as possible.

Type-II diabetes, also called "adult-onset" diabetes, is a more gradual process. It's as if the electric fan is slowing down and isn't able to cool the house no matter how much the thermostat tells it to.

In the early stages of Type-II diabetes, the body usually continues to produce some of its own insulin. Often, the problem is that the insulin is simply not doing its job of transporting sugar from the bloodstream into the body's cells. Often, this is caused by excess body fat, which seems to keep insulin from working at full strength. Initial treatment of Type-II diabetes usually involves exercise and weight reduction. However, as the disease progresses, the pancreas gradually wears down, and insulin injections or medications to lower blood sugar levels may be required.

Short-Term Effects

In the short-term, uncontrolled diabetes (high and low blood sugar levels) can interfere with many aspects of daily living. High blood sugar levels cause frequent urination, which can cause dehydration and affect work and sleep patterns. It can also cause muscle loss, blurred vision, insatiable thirst, irritability, muscle cramps, weakness, and a high risk of infections.

Low blood sugar, which can occur when taking insulin or certain types of diabetes pills, can cause profuse sweating, dizziness, shaking, confusion or loss of consciousness.

Long-Term Effects

Have you ever spilled a sweet drink? Makes a sticky mess, doesn't it? Excess sugar in the bloodstream causes a sticky mess as well. Sugar tends to stick to chemicals in the blood, changing them so that they damage different organs in the body.

KEY DEFINITION:

<u>Glycosylation</u> is the process by which glucose connects chemically with other substances in the body.

Diabetes is the fifth leading cause of death in the United States. It is the leading cause of blindness and one of the leading causes of kidney failure and limb amputation. Elevated blood sugar levels during pregnancy contribute to a variety of birth defects and increase the risk of miscarriage <u>four</u> <u>times</u>. The estimated cost of diabetes per year is over 110 billion dollars, which represents 12% of the total health care costs in the U.S.

But rather than dwell on the negative, from now on let's focus on what we can do to prevent the complications and thoroughly enjoy life. Remember, diabetes control does not mean being "Mr. or Ms. Perfect Patient" all the time. It means learning all we can about diabetes and making smart choices about how we live with it.

Key Point:

Understanding the truth about diabetes is the first step toward managing it successfully.

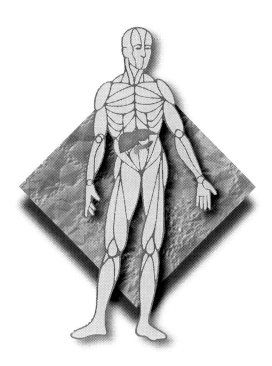

Chapter 2: Type I Diabetes

Last weekend, we took a trip to the ice cream parlor. You know, the one with 33 zillion flavors. Yours truly ordered old-fashioned strawberry. The kids wanted some kind of weird new flavor - triple berry float. The names were as different as night and day, but you know what? They both tasted about the same.

Diabetes only comes in a few flavors. The most common types, which we will discuss in this and the next chapter, are called "Type I" and "Type II" diabetes. They represent very different forms of the disease. But you know what? In terms of the symptoms people experience, they both taste about the same. Both cause blood sugar levels to go high because of a problem with the body's own natural insulin. Both require careful management of blood sugar levels. And both can cause a wide range of health problems (complications).

However, the similarities stop there. From a physiological standpoint, Type I and Type II are as different as, well, chocolate and vanilla. First lets look at the chocolate, er... Type I... diabetes.

Definition

Type-I diabetes, for lack of a better definition, means a complete lack of insulin. Insulin is produced by an organ called the pancreas, which sits just under the stomach. There are groups of cells in the pancreas called "Beta Cells". These are the cells responsible for detecting blood sugar levels and producing insulin whenever the blood sugar goes up.

> **Insulin:**
> **A hormone (natural chemical) that lowers blood sugar levels by helping get sugar from the bloodstream into the body's cells.**

In Type-I diabetes, the beta cells are destroyed, leaving the pancreas unable to make insulin. As a result, the blood sugar goes up. People with Type-I diabetes depend on insulin injections to bring the blood sugar down. Without insulin injections, the body's cells would not get the fuel they need to burn for energy, and the person would eventually die. For this reason, Type-I is also called Insulin Dependent diabetes - the person depends on insulin injections to live.

Presently, there are approximately <u>800,000</u> people in the United States with Type-I diabetes, with about <u>20,000</u> new cases added every year. Type-I diabetes usually occurs at a young age, rarely after age 30. It occurs most commonly around age 11-14, and thus the name Juvenile Diabetes is sometimes used. However, Type-I diabetes can also occur in very young children as well as teenagers and young adults.

Regardless of the age at which it starts, Type-I diabetes always means that the pancreas is no longer producing insulin.

The Causes

The process by which beta cells are destroyed is called <u>autoimmune disease</u>. Normally, our body's immune system creates soldiers (white blood cells and antibodies) that hunt down invaders like bacteria, leaving our body's own cells unharmed. In an autoimmune disease, these "soldiers" can't tell the good guys from the bad guys. They start attacking our own cells, leading to diseases such as Lupus, rheumatoid arthritis, and you guessed it, Type-I diabetes.

Beta Cells:
Cells of the pancreas that detect blood sugar levels and produce insulin.

Islet Cells:
Groups of cells in the pancreas that include beta cells.

Type-I diabetes is caused by a combination of autoimmune problems, including:

1. <u>Islet Cell Antibodies</u> - Sometimes, the immune system accidentally produces antibodies ("chemical soldiers") that destroy the beta cells of the pancreas, which are part of clusters of cells called islet cells. These Islet Cell Antibodies are present in about 75% of people with newly diagnosed Type-I diabetes.

2. <u>Insulin Autoantibodies</u> - The immune system or white blood cells may also produce antibodies that seek out and destroy insulin after it has been produced. Insulin autoantibodies are present in almost 50% of people with newly diagnosed Type-I diabetes.

3. <u>GAD</u> (Glutamic Acid Decorboxylase) Antibodies - The Beta cells produce special proteins called GAD. The immune system produces antibodies that target GAD, and ends up destroying beta cells as well. These antibodies are present in almost all the people with Type I diabetes at the time of diagnosis. Often children who acquire Coxsackie virus start producing antibodies that attack GAD in Beta cells suggesting that this common virus may be a "trigger" for autoimmune destruction of beta cells in some people.

A Chance to See Into The Future?

Antibodies such as islet cell antibodies, insulin autoantibodies, and GAD antibodies appear long before the actual destruction of Beta Cells. The major damage to beta cells is caused by white blood cells (also called T-cells or Killer Cells) that may be produced months or years after the antibodies first appear.

Thus, the presence of antibodies gives us a chance to see whether a person is susceptible to developing Type-I diabetes at a later date. For example, the brother of a girl with Type-I diabetes can be tested for islet cell antibodies to see if he is likely to develop diabetes in the future. Presently, many clinics are studying the effectiveness of different treatments aimed at slowing auto-immune destruction of beta cells and (hopefully) preventing Type 1 diabetes.

Symptoms

Just before diagnosis, a person with Type-I diabetes will likely have a very high blood sugar level and will be producing little or no insulin. As a result, the following symptoms usually occur:

1. <u>You pee a lot</u>. The kidneys try to get rid of the excess sugar through the urine, and sugar tends to drag a lot of fluid with it!

2. <u>You drink a lot</u>. With all that peeing comes a mighty powerful thirst!

3. <u>Your pants fall down</u>. Since you can't use sugar for fuel, the body starts breaking down lots of fat and protein, and rapid weight loss usually occurs.

4. <u>You have the hunger of many men (or women)</u>. Because your body is starving for energy, it cranks up the hunger sensations big time!

5. <u>You become a breeding ground for infections</u>. Due to high sugar content of the blood and other body fluids, there may be frequent vaginal infections and/or urinary tract infections (bacteria like sugar!). Sores may be slow to heal. The white blood cells that usually fight infection are bathed in sugar and can't put up a very good fight.

Sounds pretty attractive, doesn't it? Just the kind of person you might want to meet in a singles bar.

Unfortunately, many people don't recognize these symptoms in time. If the body is forced to go very long without insulin, it will usually start to break down things we need (like muscle and vital organs). When this happens, we start to produce dangerous chemical waste products called "ketone bodies". If enough ketone bodies are produced, they can make us violently ill or even cause a coma. This is called "diabetic ketoacidosis" - a subject that we will discuss in greater detail at other points throughout this book.

Key point:

Type I diabetes is usually caused by an autoimmune condition that stops the pancreas from producing insulin. Insulin injections are required to live.

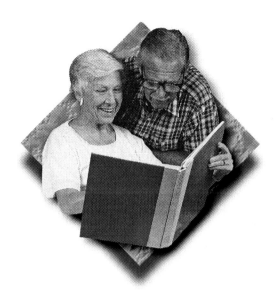

Chapter 3: Type II Diabetes

Diabetes is definitely <u>not</u> a democratic disease. How can you tell? Simple. In a democracy, the majority rules. But diabetes is ruled by the minority - the young people smitten with Type-I diabetes. When was the last time you saw a commercial or a poster about diabetes that featured an old, fat person with Type II diabetes? It's always some adorable child bemoaning the pain of daily insulin injections.

If Type-I represents the "glitz and glamour" of diabetes, then Type-II represents the heart and soul. Of the 16 million Americans who have diabetes, about 15 million have Type-II. Unlike people with Type-I, who must take insulin just to stay alive, most people with Type-II still produce some insulin on their own. They may end up taking insulin to keep the blood sugar under control, but insulin is usually not necessary for basic survival.

Why does Type-II happen?

To understand what causes Type-II diabetes, let's go back to the basics on how insulin works.

After eating, much of the food is digested into glucose, a simple sugar that circulates in the blood. For the body's cells to use glucose as a source of energy, the glucose must enter the cells through special locked doors that can only be opened with insulin "keys". Without insulin, the doors remain locked and glucose cannot enter the cells.

Insulin Resistance:
A condition in which insulin's normal blood-sugar-lowering action is reduced. More insulin than usual is required to keep blood sugar levels under control.

As people age and gain weight, insulin's job becomes tougher. There are fewer doors on the body's cells, so the insulin has to hunt down doors to unlock. Sometimes, the locks are of poor quality, and the insulin keys don't fit quite right. Or, the key fits the lock, but the doors are stuck, and sugar cannot enter. As a result, sugar tends to build up in the blood, waiting for insulin to unlock the doors and let them into the body's cells.

In a person without diabetes, the blood sugar is maintained at a normal level of 70-120 by the pancreas, which makes enough insulin to open enough doors to get the sugar out of the bloodstream and into the cells. However, some people who are overweight have high levels of insulin in their blood. High insulin levels can cause weight gain and may be linked to complications such as high blood pressure and heart disease.

In people who are genetically prone to have diabetes (see the following section, "Who Is At Risk?"), the pancreas is unable to produce enough insulin to keep blood sugar levels from going too high. At first, a person might experience high blood sugar after meals, as the pancreas can't make insulin quickly enough to match the glucose rise from the food just eaten. This is called **Postprandial Hyperglycemia**.

Later, a person might experience high blood sugar in the early morning. This is called **Fasting Hyperglycemia**. This occurs when there isn't enough insulin to keep the liver from releasing sugar into the bloodstream just before we wake up. Remember, insulin lowers blood sugar in two ways: by packing sugar into cells, and by keeping certain cells (such as liver cells) from releasing sugar into the blood stream.

Who's At Risk?

Type-II diabetes is caused by a combination of genetic and lifestyle factors. While we can't choose our parents (although some of us wish we could), we can control many of the factors that pertain to our lifestyle. Below are the most common factors that cause Type-II diabetes:

1. Obesity

We all have a picture in our minds of a person who is obese. It may be a circus freak who weighs as much as a circus elephant. Or it may be a poor, grossly overweight individual who appeared on a TV talk show to complain about the size of airplane seats.

These represent the most extreme cases of obesity. Obesity, defined as being more than 20% over ideal body weight, is present in epidemic proportions in the United States. 35 million Americans are obese.

People who are obese are prone to developing diabetes because they are insulin resistant and require more insulin than usual to control blood sugar levels. In fact, more than 80% (4 out of 5) people with Type-II diabetes are obese. Those who have upper body obesity - thin arms and legs but a large belly - are especially susceptible to diabetes. The longer a person is overweight, and the more obese they are, the greater the chances for developing Type-II diabetes.

Are you overweight? Obese?
Do the math, and FIND OUT!

- For most adults (i.e. non-athletes/bodybuilders), ideal body weight can be figured as follows:

- Men: 106 lbs. for the first five feet of height, plus 6 lbs. for each inch above 5 ft.

- Women: 100 lbs. for the first five feet of height, plus or minus 5 lbs. for each inch above or below 5 ft.

- For example, Gertrude is 5 feet 3 inches tall, and weighs 145 lbs. Her ideal body weight is 100 (for the first 5 feet), plus 15 (for the additional 3 inches), or 115 lbs.

- To figure her percent over ideal body weight, divide the actual weight by the ideal weight and subtract 1. 145/115 = 1.26, minus 1 = .26.

- Gertrude is 26% over ideal body weight. She is obese.

2. Age

This falls under the category of "stuff we can't do a thing about".

As we age, we tend to develop more body fat, lose some muscle, and have a weaker pancreas than we had at a younger age. Above age 40, the risk of Type-II diabetes goes up significantly.

3. Family History

The tendency to develop Type-II diabetes is often inherited. If any of your blood relatives have Type-II diabetes, you may have the "weak pancreas" gene that puts you at risk for Type-II diabetes as well.

Statistics show that a person has a 35% chance of developing Type-II diabetes if one parent has it. If both parents have diabetes, the risk rises to 70%. If this person becomes obese, it is very likely that he or she will develop Type-II diabetes.

Why don't all children of diabetic parents go on to develop diabetes? Because the only thing that is inherited is a tendency to develop diabetes, not diabetes itself. Countless people who have the tendency but take good care of themselves (i.e. eat right, exercise, control their weight) never go on to develop diabetes.

4. Complications from Pregacy

A woman who: (A) developed gestational diabetes during pregnancy, (B) gave birth to a child weighing more than 9 lbs., or (C) had a still birth runs a high risk of developing Type-II diabetes later in life.

5. Ethnicity

Certain ethnic groups, including Native Americans, African Americans, and Hispanic Americans are at a high risk for developing Type-II diabetes (see chart below).

Percentage with Diabetes by Ethnicity

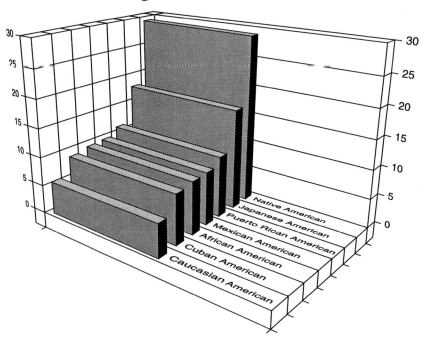

6. Inactivity

Inactive people have a higher than average risk of developing diabetes. Exercise helps a person to lose weight, and makes insulin more effective. The more calories burned per week though exercise, the lower a person's risk of developing Type-II diabetes.

7. Presence of Other Health Problems

Bad news comes in bunches. People who already have high blood pressure (greater than 140/90), high cholesterol (over 200) or high triglycerides (over 150) are more likely to develop Type-II diabetes.

A Progressive Illness

Calling Type-II diabetes a progressive illness does not mean that it is hip, cool or modern. We'll reserve that kind of talk for things like art and music.

Type-II diabetes is progressive because it starts small and grows worse, like a snowball rolling down a steep hill.

In the earliest stages of Type-II diabetes, the blood sugar may be perfectly normal. However, the pancreas is working overtime to produce enough extra insulin to keep the sugar within normal range. This is called the stage of **insulin resistance**.

Once insulin resistance sets in, it may take 10 years or longer before blood sugar levels begin rising above normal. In some cases, high blood sugar is first detected during routine insurance exams or company physicals, or during hospitalization for a completely different condition.

The second stage of diabetes is called **impaired glucose tolerance.** By definition, it means fasting plasma sugar (blood sugar first thing in the morning) of 110-140, or blood sugar between 140 and 200 two hours after a meal. Some doctors refer to this as "a touch of diabetes". We refer to it as "your last chance to get in shape before full-blown diabetes sets in." It is at this "critical point" that your body has become so insulin resistant that your pancreas just can't make enough insulin to keep the blood sugar under control. Change your habits and lose weight now, and you may be able to bring your sugar down and keep your pancreas from burning itself out. Keep on doing what you're doing, and higher blood sugar - and the diagnosis of diabetes - is just around the corner.

By definition, **diabetes** means that you have fasting blood sugars over 140, or after-meal blood sugars over 200. Many of the symptoms are similar to those that occur in Type-I diabetes. These are caused by high blood sugar levels:

- Frequent Urination

- Increased Thirst

- Blurred Vision

- Vaginal or Urinary Tract Infections

- Dry, itchy skin

Because the symptoms of Type-II diabetes are slow to develop and may be mild, a person could have Type-II for many years without being diagnosed or treated. For that reason, long-term complications of diabetes (heart disease, nerve disease, eye disease, kidney damage, poor circulation in the legs and feet) may be present at the time Type-II diabetes is first diagnosed. In fact, at the time of diagnosis, people with Type-II diabetes also have heart disease 50% of the time, eye damage 20% of the time, and poor circulation in the legs 8% of the time.

Treatment of Type-II Diabetes

To treat Type-II diabetes means more than just keeping the blood sugar levels as close to normal as possible. It also means controlling total cholesterol levels, HDLs/LDLs (High Density Lipoproteins /Low Density Lipoproteins), triglycerides, blood pressure, and obesity. The goal of all this is to prevent the complications of diabetes (including heart attack, stroke, kidney failure, blindness and foot amputation), and live not only a long life, but a high quality life.

Our arsenal of weapons for controlling blood sugar in Type-II diabetes includes a healthy diet, exercise, and possibly oral medications or insulin.

Diet is a four-letter word in most circles. Better to think of it as good, healthy eating. If you think a "diabetic diet" means no sweets, you must still be living in the 1950s. We now know that a "diabetic diet" is the same healthy nutrition plan that all Americans are encouraged to follow: Plenty of complex carbohydrates, moderate amounts of protein, increased fiber and low salt. Fats should be eaten sparingly due to their high calorie content. Whenever possible, monounsaturated and polyunsaturated fats (from plant sources) should be used in place of saturated fats (from animal sources). This will help to increase the "good cholesterol" (HDL) and lower the "bad cholesterol" (LDL). Diet will be discussed in greater detail in chapter 4.

Weight loss is also a major part of the treatment of Type-II diabetes. Why? Because modest weight loss helps overcome insulin resistance and bring blood sugar levels down. As you will read in chapter 16, weight loss requires you to burn more calories than you take in. That means reducing total calorie intake, and increasing your calorie expenditure through **exercise**.

Exercise serves multiple purposes for people with Type-II diabetes. Besides helping you to lose weight, exercise provides an immediate reduction in blood sugar. When done consistently, exercise can also help to prevent long-term complications such as heart disease and stroke.

Exercise and a low-calorie, healthy diet are the cornerstones of managing Type-II diabetes. Too often, doctors ignore these basic treatments in favor of pills or insulin because they don't require as much work. But are they better for you? Hardly.

Most **diabetes pills** (sulfonylureas or OHAs - oral hypoglycemic agents) lower blood sugar by making the pancreas produce more insulin. While this may work in some cases, it can also cause additional weight gain. People with Type-II diabetes gain an average of 3-6 lbs. when taking an OHA, and 11-22 lbs. when taking insulin. And more importantly, they fail to correct the root of the problem: insulin resistance.

So, THE FIRST ORDER OF BUSINESS IN TREATING TYPE-II DIABETES IS WEIGHT LOSS. This may require that you work with a dietitian and possibly an exercise physiologist. But if you value your health, it is well worth the effort.

Some of the newer medications for controlling blood sugar, Glucophage (metformin) and Precose (acarbose), do not cause weight gain, unlike OHAs and insulin. However, they do not work in all cases. Glucophage and Precose can be started at any time - with diet/exercise, or after. OHAs should only be used after weight loss fails to bring the blood sugar levels down.

For some people, permanent weight loss helps to control Type-II diabetes indefinitely. However, if weight loss and diabetes pills fail to do the job, insulin injections become necessary. Even if diabetes pills seem to do the job for a while, their effectiveness usually fades over time.

Approximately 30% of people with Type-II diabetes take insulin. Remember, this does not mean that they now have Type-I diabetes. They are simply considered to have Type-II diabetes that is controlled with the aid of insulin.

The Big Misconceptions

Here are a few of the common misconceptions concerning Type-II diabetes:

1. Doctors are weight loss experts.

Historically, doctors don't do a very good job helping their patients lose weight. Ninety percent of people with Type-II diabetes <u>do</u> <u>not</u> lose weight, and wind up needing pills or insulin to control their diabetes. Unless you are seeing a doctor who specializes in weight control or metabolic disorders, you are going to need some outside help. Dietitians, group exercise classes and weight loss programs may provide the push and direction you need.

2. Type-II diabetes isn't that serious.

Many people with Type-II diabetes think that their disease is not all that bad, especially if they don't take insulin. This false sense of security keeps them from losing weight and doing the right things to control the disease. The fact is, Type II diabetes is like a pit bull: DEADLY if not treated properly. Often, Type-II diabetes is accompanied by high blood pressure, high cholesterol, high triglycerides and obesity. The result: the person with Type-II diabetes is a breeding ground for circulatory problems, which usually lead to heart attack, stroke, and foot/leg amputation.

3. Insulin solves the problem.

True, insulin is the quick fix for high blood sugar. But insulin may create more problems than it solves.

Insulin stimulates the appetite and causes the body's cells to absorb more nutrients, which cause weight gain. Weight gain creates insulin resistance, which means that more insulin is needed. More insulin starts the cycle all over again. And don't forget, insulin can cause low blood sugar (hypoglycemia) if meals are not eaten in a timely and appropriate manner. In fact, the risk of hypoglycemia is so great in some elderly people that it may be safer to run blood sugars that are a little on the high side rather than within the normal range.

4. Once you have Type-II diabetes, it can't get any worse.

If you have diabetes and don't do the right things to control it (like losing weight), things are definitely going to get worse. You will probably wind up taking a whole slew of medications for things like blood pressure, cholesterol, poor circulation, and infection. You will probably wind up taking insulin, because your pancreas becomes burned out from overproduction. You will also probably suffer from poor circulation as high blood sugar makes things "sticky" in the bloodstream. Not surprisingly, the most common cause of death in Type-II diabetes is heart disease.

5. There's no rush to get diabetes under control.

Every day your blood sugar levels are elevated, every day you are carrying too much weight, every day your blood pressure or cholesterol are too high, your circulation is becoming worse and worse. Most of the damage that occurs (narrowing and hardening of the arteries) is not reversible. Deal with your diabetes today, because you may not have a chance tomorrow.

Picture This

August 6, 1986:

Milton went for a physical exam because he was going to the bathroom all night long. His doctor diagnosed Type-II diabetes, and told Milton that he should try to lose weight. He also gave Milton a pill to take (an oral hypoglycemic agent), and asked him to come back next month for another blood sugar check.

Milton didn't worry too much about having diabetes. Then, two days before his appointment, he started to experience chest pains. He was rushed to the hospital, where he was told that he had a mild heart attack. His blood sugar was so high that he was put on insulin injections twice a day. He was also scheduled for angioplasty to help open the blood vessels leading to his heart.

Milton never got off of insulin injections. To this day, he suffers from heart disease and poor circulation in his legs which causes him tremendous pain at night and keeps him at home most of the time.

August 6, 1996:

Mabel went to her doctor because she was feeling weak and was constantly thirsty and going to the bathroom. Her doctor diagnosed her with Type-II diabetes, and warned her about how serious it could be. He told her that her blood sugar was very high, but it could come down if she lost weight. Mabel was taught how to check her own blood sugar, and was scheduled for a follow-up appointment in one month.

The next day, Mabel went to see a dietitian, who helped her design a sensible meal plan. She learned that she could eat healthy and cut calories without feeling hungry. She also started exercising each morning. She noticed that her blood sugar was better after exercising and following her meal plan.

At her next visit, the doctor weighed Mabel. She had lost eight pounds and her blood sugar was beginning to come down. The doctor said, "Mabel, you're doing a great job. Keep it up, and you can keep your diabetes under control without pills or insulin."

Mabel was so proud that she bought herself a new pair of walking shoes. She plans to walk with her grandchildren to raise funds for diabetes research in the fall.

Key Point:

The first order of business in managing Type-II diabetes is immediate and permanent weight loss.

Section II

Tools of the Trade

These days, everyone has their own tools. Doctors have their medical instruments. Chefs have their lucky spatulas. Computer gurus have their bytes and rams and gigathingamajigs.

People with diabetes have their own set of weapons for doing battle in the blood sugar wars. They are: healthy food, exercise, and insulin/oral medications. These will be covered in detail in this section. The thing that ties them together is blood glucose monitoring and the ability to make intelligent decisions regarding day-to-day control. This will be the topic of Section III.

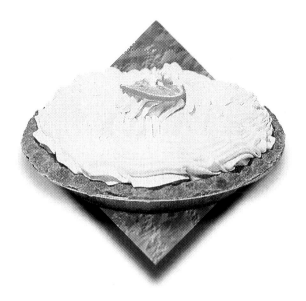

Chapter 4: There Is No "Diabetic Diet"

Every year, Steve goes home for the holidays. As he approaches the house, the smell of fresh pies, breads and pastries fills the air. After he opens the door and shares a smattering of hugs and kisses, he starts edging his way toward the dessert table, thinking to himself, "This year, I'm actually going to make it. Nothing can stop me now!"

Suddenly, Aunt Alice plants herself squarely between Steve and the desserts, sporting a bright red beehive hairdo and a bowl of green sugar-free gelatin laced with tiny banana slices.

"Now don't you go near that table," she says in a deep voice, the kind you get from smoking cigarettes for a thousand years. "I made this just for you. I'm always looking out for my Stevie!"

"Aunt Alice, you know I can eat the same things as everyone else."

"Oh, nonsense. We all know that diabetics shouldn't have sugar. It'll make you go blind."

Blind with rage, maybe. What Aunt Alice fails to understand is that people with diabetes can eat just about anything and as much or as little as they choose. It's all a matter of compensating with our other weapons - exercise, insulin and diabetes medications — so that the blood sugar does not go too high or low.

Aunt Alice isn't the only one who is misinformed. The traditional "diabetic diet" that many doctors still hand to their patients just serve to confuse and alienate. The term "diet" itself can be a depressing word. The concept of "meal planning" is a bit easier to grasp and not quite as intimidating.

The recommended meal plan for most people with diabetes is the same as the dietary guidelines for all Americans set by the American Heart Association and American Cancer Society. It is something that the whole family can use. With the guidance of a qualified diabetes educator, everyone with diabetes should gain an understanding of how to balance different foods with their insulin, medications, and exercise.

Why is meal planning important?

Proper meal planning is important for everyone. For those with diabetes, it is the cornerstone of good control.

Food provides the calories (energy) that are needed to keep us alive and physically active. Food also supplies the minerals and nutrients necessary for bodily growth, repair, and good health.

The meal plan can be tailored to allow us to gain weight, lose weight, or maintain weight. This is based on an individual's calorie consumption and requirements, a subject that will be discussed in greater detail later in this chapter.

Meal planning can be used to reduce the risk of heart attack, stroke and other circulatory problems. By reducing intake of fats (especially saturated fats), it is possible to maintain cholesterol and triglyceride levels within a normal range. Limiting sodium (salt) intake can help to control blood pressure. Dietary intake of certain minerals can improve blood sugar control and lower the risk for heart disease. These too will be discussed later in this chapter.

Finally, meal planning is essential for good blood sugar control. Those taking insulin or oral hypoglycemic agents (diabetes pills) must time meals and snacks carefully to avoid low blood sugar. Planning meals and snacks with consistent amounts of carbohydrate will enhance blood sugar control. Generally, it is also better to have many small meals and snacks than just a few large meals. That way, rises and falls in blood sugar will be modest rather than severe.

Food for thought: Background Information

There are three different energy sources found in most foods: Carbohydrate (which includes sugar and starch), Protein, and Fat. Most foods contain a combination of these energy sources, along with vitamins, minerals, and fiber.

CARBOHYDRATES

When food is digested, all of the carbohydrates (whether they were in the form of simple sugars or starches) are converted into glucose, the sugar that is transported in the bloodstream. A cup of rice containing 45 grams of carbohydrate will raise the blood sugar just as much as a can of regular, sugar-sweetened soda which also contains 45 grams of carbohydrate. The blood sugar will usually rise a few minutes after eating food high in carbohydrates, and will reach its highest point 60-90 minutes after a meal.

Foods rich in carbohydrate include sweets, fruits and juices, breads, cereals, rice, beans, and starchy vegetables like corn and potatoes. In terms of calorie content, carbohydrates are relatively "light". Every gram of carbohydrate contains just four calories. Thus, a slice of bread that contains 15 grams of carbohydrate also contains 4X15, or 60 calories.

PROTEIN

Some of the protein we eat is converted into sugar. However, this conversion takes a long time, and only a small portion of the protein is actually turned into sugar. For example, an 8-ounce steak may cause a modest rise in blood sugar several hours after it is eaten, whereas a baked potato may cause a sharp rise in blood sugar 30 minutes after it is eaten.

Foods high in protein include beef, poultry, fish, eggs, nuts, and milk products. Each gram of protein contains four calories - the same amount as carbohydrate.

FAT

Only a small portion of fat is converted to sugar, and this may take several hours to occur. In other words, the immediate impact of fat on blood sugar levels is very small.

Every gram of fat contains nine calories - more than twice as much as protein and carbohydrate. A high-fat diet often leads to weight gain, and extra body fat keeps insulin from doing its job properly. As a result, a high-fat, high-calorie diet can impair blood sugar control over the long-term.

There are also three different types of fat: monounsaturated, polyunsaturated, and saturated. We like to call them the good, the bad and the ugly. "Mono" fats tend to lower the blood cholesterol level; "poly" tends to keep them about the same; and saturated fat tends to raise it. All three have the same high calorie content and contribute to weight gain.

THE CALORIE CONNECTION

Calories are really just units of energy, just like gasoline is energy for a car. If we fill up a gas tank, the car has plenty of energy to go where it needs to. If we over-fill the tank, the extra gas has to go someplace; usually it spills all over our hands and feet.

Likewise, if we take in more calories than we burn up, the extra calories have to go somewhere. You guessed it - they get stored as body fat. The fat will only get used up if we start to burn more calories than we take in. It doesn't matter where the calories came from, whether it be carbohydrates, proteins, or fats in our diet. Eat more than you burn, and you gain weight. Burn more than you eat, and you lose weight.

Calories are burned in two ways: through physical activity such as exercise and daily chores, and by our basic metabolism which just serves to keep us alive (heart beating, eyes blinking, etc.).

DESIRABLE BODY WEIGHT 5'6" = 130#

For women: 100 lbs. for first 5 feet tall, plus 5 lbs.
for each extra inch tall.

For men: 106 lbs. for first 5 feet tall, plus 6 lbs. 6'1" = 184#
for each extra inch tall.

Here is a simple formula for figuring out how many calories you burn each day:

If you are sedentary most of the time, multiply your desirable body weight in pounds (DBW) times 10 if you are a woman, or by 13 if you are a man. If you lead an active lifestyle, multiply your desirable body weight by 15, and add any calories you burn exercising.

For example, a 5-foot, 2-inch woman who walks two miles a day burns 1850 calories:

$$DBW = 100 + 2X5 = 110$$

$$110 \text{ X } 15 = 1650 \text{ calories, plus } 200 \text{ exercise calories} = 1850$$
$$\text{calories/day}$$

If you are overweight and your doctor has advised you to lose weight, you can do so through a sensible plan that involves reducing your total caloric intake and increasing your caloric expenditure.

To lose body fat, you must burn more calories than you take in. This is called a "calorie deficit" in honor of our Federal Government which has been spending more than it takes in for years. It takes a 3500 calorie deficit to burn one pound of fat.

Reducing your calorie intake usually involves reducing the amount of fat in the diet, and carefully reducing the portion sizes of foods you like to eat. You can burn more calories by exercising and raising your body's metabolism, which takes place through muscle growth. These will be discussed in greater detail in Chapter 16.

Approaches to meal planning: A menu of choices

There are a number of approaches to meal planning, each with its own benefits and drawbacks.

1. The Food Guide Pyramid

According to the food guide pyramid, healthy eating means having a balanced diet that gives your body what it needs, and minimizing those things that you can do without.

According to the pyramid, grains, beans and starchy foods supply carbohydrates for energy, and should be the staple of your meal plan. Fruits and vegetables supply essential vitamins, minerals and fiber and are low in calories. Milk and meat products supply the protein necessary for bodily growth and repair, and help promote all the biochemical reactions that keep us alive and healthy. However, meat and milk products are also high in fat and calories. Since the body needs only a small amount of protein each day, milk and meat products should be consumed in modest amounts. Fats, sweets and alcohol provide "empty" calories. They contribute to weight gain without supplying vitamins, minerals, protein and fiber, and should be consumed as little as possible.

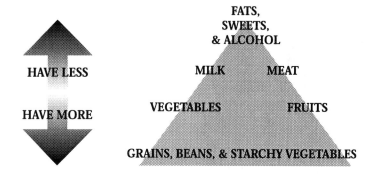

THE FOOD GUIDE PYRAMID

The pyramid concept is simple to understand, and is on target in terms of providing adequate nutrition without including too much of the bad stuff in the diet. Perhaps the biggest drawback to the Food Guide Pyramid is that it is not individualized. It does not consider a person's caloric needs or weight gain/loss needs. It also does not take into account the effects different foods have on blood sugar levels. A meal plan that contains an excess of fruits and starches will ultimately lead to high blood sugar and increased insulin needs.

2. Sample Menus

Many brochures and books provide sample meals that are designed specifically for managing diabetes and/or losing weight. These typically include recipes for low-fat foods with the quantities specified in order to control the amount of carbohydrates and calories that are being consumed. Obviously, sample menus can benefit anyone who wants clear, specific direction. However, what it offers in precision, it lacks in flexibility. Real-life often calls for dining out - at parties, friends' homes, family holiday meals, and at restaurants.

3. Exchange Systems (Food Choices)

You may have heard people with diabetes saying that they get "three breads at breakfast, four at lunch, four at dinner, and two at bedtime." Maybe that explains why the supermarket is always out of bread when you show up.

A "bread" does not necessarily mean a slice of bread. It means a food item that is similar in carbohydrate, fat and protein content to a slice of bread. A slice of bread has mostly carbohydrate (15 grams per serving), with a small amount of protein and fat. The same can be said for half a cup of spaghetti, three cups of air-popped popcorn, one very small potato, or 1/3 cup of corn. In other words, three cups of popcorn can be "exchanged" for a slice of bread because it contains about the same nutrients.

The same can be said for the other exchanges. A meat exchange contains a lot of protein, a moderate-to-high amount of fat, and very little carbohydrate - just like a typical piece of meat. You could call it a "purple" exchange if you wanted to, but calling it a meat exchange reminds us of the kind of nutrients it contains.

Below is the general content of the different exchange groups, per serving:

Exchange Group	Examples	Carbohydrate	Protein	Fat
Bread	1 slice Bread 3/4 cup Corn flakes 1/2 cup Noodles 6 saltine Crackers	Lots (15g)	Little (3g)	Little (1g)
Fruit	1/2 cup Orange juice 1/2 Banana 1 small Apple 1 cup Watermelon	Lots (15g)	None (0g)	None (0g)
Vegetable	1/3 cup cooked Carrots 1/2 cup fresh Peas 1 cup Spinach 1/2 cup canned Tomato	Little (5g)	Little (2g)	None (0g)
Milk	1 cup Milk 1/2 cup Ice Cream	Moderate (12g)	Lots (8g)	Varies (1-8g)
Meat	1 oz. Meat 1 oz. Cheese 1 oz. Sandwich meat	None (0g)	Lots (7g)	Varies (3-8g)
Fat	1 tsp. Butter 1 strip Bacon 1 tsp. Vegetable oil 2 tbs. Sour cream	None (0g)	None (0g)	Lots (5g)

The exchange diet is beneficial for people with diabetes because it specifies the amount of fat, protein and carbohydrate in the meal plan, and builds in a great deal of variety. The total calorie level usually determines the quantities of the different exchanges, and the number of meals and snacks. However, the exchange system is complex and cumbersome, and takes a long time to master. It may be difficult to follow when eating away from home. There also tends to be a great deal of confusion regarding the precise quantity of food that makes up a particular exchange.

4. Counting Systems: Carbohydrates, Fat Grams, and Calories

Counting systems are really just simplified versions of the exchange systems, focusing on one particular aspect of the meal plan.

Calorie counting involves simply adding up total calorie intake throughout the day. It is critical to understand portion sizes when counting calories, as this has a significant impact on calorie consumption. Calorie counting is the most direct and convenient way to monitor and reduce calorie intake, but it does not consider the impact of foods on blood sugar, and fails to specify the types of foods that are needed for healthy living.

Fat gram counting is done mainly to limit total calorie intake and lower cholesterol and triglyceride levels. By limiting total fat intake, it is possible to indirectly reduce total calorie intake and thus lose weight. However, fat gram counting fails to account for calorie intake from protein and carbohydrate sources, and does not consider the effect of different foods on blood sugar levels.

Carbohydrate counting is perhaps the most effective way to manage blood sugar levels. Remember, carbohydrates have by far the greatest impact on blood sugar, so controlling how much carbohydrate you are eating will ultimately produce the best blood sugar results.

For example, consider the following breakfasts:

Breakfast A	
Large Bowl of Cereal	(30g carb)
1 Cup 2% Milk	(12g carb)
8 oz. Orange Juice	(30g carb)
Total Carbohydrates	72 grams

Breakfast B			Breakfast C	
2 Eggs w/Bacon	(0g carb)		Small Bowl of Cereal	(20g carb)
2 Toast & Butter	(30g carb)		4 Oz. Skim Milk	(6g carb)
Coffee & Cream	(5g carb)		1/2 Banana	(15g carb)
	35grams			41 grams

Breakfast A has about twice as many carbohydrates as breakfasts B and C, and would cause the greatest rise in blood sugar. Breakfast B has the least carbohydrates, but contains more fat and calories than the other two, and would not be optimal for those trying to keep their weight under control. Breakfast C contains a modest amount of carbohydrate and is low in calories, and would probably be the best choice for someone trying to control their weight as well as their blood sugar.

Carb counting is especially useful for people who adjust their insulin doses, such as those who are taking multiple injections or using an insulin pump. More carbohydrate simply means more pre-meal insulin; less carb means less insulin. Even for those who don't take insulin or adjust their doses, carb counting allows you to have consistent blood sugars from day to day while having a variety of foods.

On the downside, carb counting requires some time to learn. Besides reading food labels, you must become good at measuring foods (on a food scale or in a measuring cup). Carb counting also neglects to account for the delayed effect of fat and protein on blood sugar levels, and it ignores the calorie content of the meal plan entirely.

The Amazing Ghani-Scheiner Meal Plan

What's good for the goose may not be good for the gander. In other words, successful meal planning requires individualization. Usually, no single approach to meal planning works all the time. The best approach is actually a combination of different approaches, based on your lifestyle, preferences, goals and abilities. It is a good idea to work with a dietitian at a local hospital or diabetes education program. See chapter 24 for more information on selecting and utilizing a dietitian.

In general, carbohydrate counting is the optimal appraoch for controlling blood sugar. No other method is as precise and simple to use as carbohydrate counting. It is easy to adjust insulin doses appropriately when you know how much carbohydrate you are going to have.

For those trying to lose weight, calorie counting may be the most practical approach. Since calories are the ultimate cause of weight gain and/or loss, counting calories is the direct route to success.

Below are some meal planning concepts that everyone can use to their advantage.

CALORIE DISTRIBUTION

The way your calories are "distributed" (i.e. what portion of your calories come from fat, protein and carbohydrate) is important for just about everyone. Approximately half of your calories should come from carbohydrates. No more than 30% should come from fat, and no more than 20% from protein. If you have kidney disease, your protein intake may need to be restricted further (see chapter 26). Remember, one gram of carb or protein has 4 calories, and one gram of fat has 9 calories. So, for a person on an 1800-calorie meal plan, the following daily totals apply:

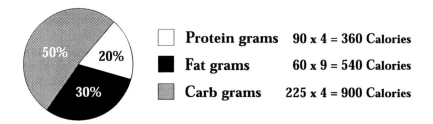

Protein grams	90 x 4 = 360 Calories
Fat grams	60 x 9 = 540 Calories
Carb grams	225 x 4 = 900 Calories

FAT SELECTION

Excessive amounts of dietary fat are responsible for heart disease, cancer, obesity and - you guessed it - Type II diabetes. For a healthy life, it is important to reduce the fat in your diet.

Remember, different types of fats have different effects on triglycerides and cholesterol levels (fats that circulate in the bloodstream). Our goal is to reduce the amount of triglycerides and "bad" cholesterols (LDLs) in the blood, while increasing the amount of "good" cholesterols (HDLs).

HDL CHOLESTEROL

HDLs are substances that take fats and cholesterol out of the blood vessels and return them to the liver for processing, thereby helping to unclog the arteries.

LDL CHOLESTEROL

LDLs are cholesterol-containing substances that stick to blood vessel walls, causing narrowing of the arteries.

For starters, cholesterol in the diet is particularly harmful, and should be limited to 300 mg a day. Read your food labels! Organ meats are very high in cholesterol. One egg yolk has 225 mg cholesterol. Limit yourself to two egg yolks a week. Egg whites can be eaten freely.

Saturated fat is the kind that raises LDLs, and can lead to blockages in the arteries. Limit your intake of saturated fats as much as possible.

Saturated fat is solid at room temperature. Butter, cream, coconut oil, palm oil, gravies, cream sauces and fatty meats are loaded with saturated fat. Meats that are marbled, such as ribeyes, chuck roasts, ground beef and shoulder roasts are high in saturated fat, as are breakfast and lunch meats such as sausage and salami.

When you want to include fat in your meal plan, choose unsaturated fats (particularly monounsaturated fat). These are liquid at room temperature, and tend to increase HDLs (the "good" cholesterol). Foods high in unsaturated fats include olive oil, corn oil, safflower oil, canola oil, and nuts. In fact, consumption of monounsaturated fat may actually reduce your total cholesterol and triglycerides. But don't go overboard - all fats, including unsaturated fats, are very high in calories!

Below are some other tips for reducing the amount of unhealthy fat in your meal plan:

- Remove the skin before eating poultry. Most of the fat is in the skin.
- Choose turkey and chicken. They have less fat than duck and goose.
- Choose fish packed in water rather than oil. Salmon, sardines and mackerel are among the best fish choices.
- When pan frying or sautéing, use a non-stick pan or low-fat cooking spray rather than butter or margarine.
- When preparing vegetables, it is best to steam, stir-fry or microwave rather than prepare them in butter sauce or cream.
- Drink skim milk rather than whole milk. Reduce your intake of cream, half and half, whipped cream, sour cream, ricotta cheese, cream cheese, and hard cheeses such as Swiss, American and cheddar.
- At breakfast, stick with whole-grain cereals or oatmeal. Watch out for croissants, granolas, pastries, muffins and biscuits -they are usually high in fat.

- Low-fat deserts/snacks include sherbet, frozen yogurt, popsicles, air-popped popcorn, pretzels and fruit. Enjoy these in place of ice cream, potato chips, tortilla chips, buttered popcorn, pies, cakes and chocolate candy.

- If you cannot substitute foods (such as having turkey rather than steak), at least reduce your portion size or eat it less often.

- Extend meat dishes with beans, vegetables or pasta rather than fatty sauces.

- Jelly is lower in fat and calories than peanut butter. Try a jelly sandwich!

- Learn to read food labels. Don't be fooled by the "low fat" or "low cholesterol" slogan. Look for the grams of fat and cholesterol per serving. Remember, total cholesterol intake should be less than 300 mg per day, and total fat intake should be limited to no more than 30% of your calorie intake. If you plan to have 1200 calories a day, you should have less than 40 grams of fat per day. 1500 calories: 50 grams of fat. 1800 calories: 60 grams of fat, and so on.

For more tips, see Stomach... er, make that Appendix A: Skim the Milk and Spare the Fat: Basic Low-Fat Cooking Techniques.

DON'T FORGET FIBER

Fiber is the part of food that is not digested. There are two kinds of fiber, both of which are beneficial in modest amounts.

Water insoluble fiber, found in foods like wheat, vegetables, whole grain bread and whole grain cereals, helps to prevent constipation and add bulk to the diet. In other words, they make you feel full so you are likely to eat less than usual.

Water soluble fiber, found in fruit, seeds, oats and beans, slows and reduces the absorption of sugar and fat from the digestive tract. Including water soluble fiber in the meal plan can reduce blood sugar levels as well as fats in the blood.

Most Americans eat less than 12 grams of fiber a day. To enjoy fiber's benefits, 25-30 grams a day are recommended. This can be accomplished by:

- Having brown rice rather than white rice.
- Eating whole fruit rather than drinking fruit juice.
- Choosing whole grain breads and cereals.
- Eating 3-5 servings of vegetables each day.

Keep in mind that changing the amount of fiber in your diet suddenly can cause gas and discomfort. Increase it gradually and drink extra water to smooth the transition.

USE SNACKS TO YOUR ADVANTAGE

Snacks are not just bad habits. They can serve a useful purpose in the management of diabetes.

Mid-morning and mid-afternoon snacks can be used to avoid low blood sugar caused by morning regular or NPH/Lente insulin, respectively. These snacks should consist of mostly carbohydrate. Bedtime snacks can be used to avoid low blood sugar during the night for those who use NPH, Lente or Ultralente insulins. The bedtime snack should contain some protein along with carbohydrate to prolong its absorption.

Snacks can also help curb the mealtime appetite. A pre-meal snack that is rich in fiber, such as an apple, can allow you to reduce the size of your meal without feeling hungry.

TIMING IS (ALMOST) EVERYTHING

Remember, if you want to control diabetes, you have to think like a pancreas! A healthy pancreas releases insulin just after you eat in order to bring the blood sugar level back toward normal. Since most people with diabetes eat three meals and several snacks a day, you should consider whether or not your insulin is active at the times when your blood sugar is on the rise — namely soon after you eat.

What would happen if your pancreas released its insulin, but you hadn't just eaten? Chances are, your blood sugar would go too low, and you would become hypoglycemic. That's what can happen if you take insulin or a pill for your diabetes and don't eat at the times your doctor, nurse or dietitian recommend.

Now, what would happen if you ate a meal, and your pancreas decided to take a coffee break for a few hours and wait to release insulin? The food you just ate is being digested and your blood sugar is rising, reaching its highest point 30-90 minutes after the meal. Of course, with no insulin to bring it down, your blood sugar could go very high. That is what happens to people who take regular or NPH insulin just as they are about to eat. Even regular insulin, which is relatively fast acting, takes a half hour to start entering your blood stream, and doesn't work its hardest until two to three hours after it is injected. That's why people who take insulin should time their meals so that they are consumed 30-60 minutes after taking an injection of regular insulin.

Humalog insulin, on the other hand, works almost immediately after it is injected. If you take Humalog insulin and then wait 30 or 60 minutes to eat, you may get low blood sugar before the plate hits the table. If your blood sugar is near normal, you should eat immediately after taking Humalog insulin. If your blood sugar is on the low side, or if you are not sure of how much you are going to eat, it may be best to take Humalog after finishing your meal!

Salt: The Hidden Enemy

Salt is important to our survival. Without salt, we could not exist.

The trouble is, you can have too much of a good thing. The price we pay for having too much salt in our diets is hypertension (high blood pressure).

It isn't just the salt shaker that we have to be concerned about. A great deal of salt is in our food before we ever reach for the shaker. Our fast food industry, for example, is notorious for using huge amounts of salt, because that's what sells.

Consider this: the recommended daily intake of sodium (the most common form of salt used in foods) is 1000 to 3000 mg per day. A single piece of fried chicken contains 500 to 1000 mg of sodium, as does a typical fast food hamburger. A single Italian sub sandwich already exceeds 3000 mg of sodium.

The typical American diet includes 5000 to 10,000 mg sodium per day. That is why hypertension (high blood pressure) is so common. High salt intake puts a great deal of strain on the kidneys. Over a period of time it can lead to dangerously high blood pressure levels (above 140/90).

The good news is that hypertension is very easy to diagnose and treat. Exercise and weight loss can lower blood pressure, and there are some excellent medications to treat it as well.

The bad news is that uncontrolled hypertension is downright deadly. Stroke, heart attack, kidney failure, blindness and hardening of the arteries are the price we pay for uncontrolled hypertension.

Aside from fast food, foods that tend to be very high in sodium include:

- Lunch meats: hot dogs, ham, bologna, salami
- Condiments: Dressings, sauces, catsup, and meat tenderizer
- Cured foods: pickles, bacon, deli meats
- Ethnic dishes: Chinese and Mexican foods
- Canned and frozen foods
- Chips and dips
- Cheeses

Here are a few tips for limiting the amount of sodium in your meal plan:

1. Try to cook your own food from scratch.
2. Read food labels; know the sodium content of the foods you commonly eat. Don't be misled. "No added salt" does not mean sodium-free.
3. Enhance flavor with lemon, onion, garlic or spices rather than salt.
4. Avoid Caesar salads. Choose vinegar and oil dressings.
5. Select foods that are broiled, baked, grilled, steamed or poached rather than sautéed or escalloped.

The Role of Chromium and Magnesium

Chromium and Magnesium are minerals that the body needs to allow our cells to function properly.

Although the exact action of chromium is not fully understood, it is believed to play a role in helping insulin carry out its primary mission: getting sugar out of the bloodstream and into the cells. The recommended daily intake of chromium is 50 to 200 micrograms for adults (1000 micrograms = 1 milligram). However, daily intake of 500 to 1000 micrograms has been shown to improve blood sugar control in many people with Type-II diabetes.

Considering that the typical American has less than 50 micrograms of chromium a day, it may be beneficial to take a chromium supplement, known as chromium picolonate. Be aware that chromium supplementation does not work for everybody, and it is not a substitute for exercise and weight control or specific diabetes medications.

Magnesium acts differently than chromium, but its effects are equally as important. Magnesium helps to open up blood vessels, which keeps the blood pressure down. Americans tend to have low levels of magnesium, mainly from eating too many processed foods and not enough foods like whole grains, beans, nuts and spinach which are naturally high in magnesium. <u>Blood levels of magnesium should be checked twice a year, and the result should be above 1.7</u>. Ask your doctor to perform this test if it is not being done already.

Uncontrolled diabetes can also lead to magnesium deficiency. Because magnesium is lost through the urine, anything that causes extra urination - including high blood sugar, diuretics (water pills) and alcohol - can lead to a magnesium shortage. Besides affecting blood pressure, low levels of magnesium can cause an irregular heartbeat and may make insulin less effective.

Key Point:
Meal planning allows you to manage your weight, blood sugar and cholesterol levels.

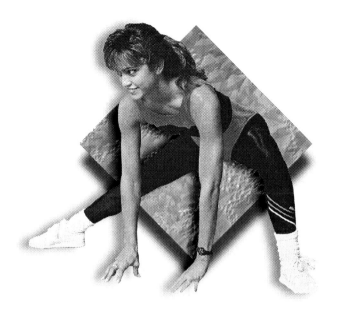

Chapter 5: Rx: Exercise

Last week, Edna made an amazing discovery that she proudly shared with her husband.

"Jim, you won't believe this, but every time I go to the mall, my blood sugar comes down. And get this - the more I spend, the more it drops!"

As you can imagine, Jim was less than thrilled to hear the news.

"Great," he said. "You mean to tell me that every time your blood sugar drops, my bank account has to drop also?"

Nobody had the heart to tell Edna that it wasn't the spending that was lowering her blood sugar. It was all the walking and package carrying she was doing. Going to the mall meant lots of walking; covering both levels meant more than a mile of walking. The more stores she entered, the more walking she did. And the more she bought, the more she wound up carrying as she walked. And the more her blood sugar would come down.

You may not think of a brisk walk, invigorating bike ride or casual game of tennis as medicine for treating your diabetes, but it is. In fact, exercise can not only help you to better manage your diabetes, it can also help to treat or offset many of the long-term complications associated with diabetes.

People with diabetes are at a high risk for heart disease, high blood pressure, infection and elevated cholesterol, as well as increased stress and a high rate of depression. Exercise is an effective, proven way to combat all of these conditions, as well as burn extra calories — an important benefit for those trying to lose weight.

As Edna discovered, exercise is also a potent tool for lowering blood sugar. It does this by improving the way insulin works.

Imagine insulin as a key that opens doors to your cells, allowing sugar to walk inside and get used for energy. Now, imagine that your cells have a sudden need for more energy. The few doors that used to be there don't allow the sugar to get in fast enough, kind of like the way traffic backs up at toll booths if there aren't enough booths open to handle all the cars.

The solution, as you might have guessed, is to open more booths. Or, in the case of your body's cells, to make more doors. Suddenly, the insulin keys have more doors to open, and sugar is able to pour out of the bloodstream and into the cells. The "traffic jam" that all that sugar was causing in the bloodstream is relieved, at least temporarily, by a single bout of exercise. Unfortunately, the extra doors built by the body's cells are only temporary; after being sedentary for a few hours, the doors get taken down and we go back to the way things were before exercising.

INSULIN SENSITIVITY

The ability of a given amount of insulin to lower the blood sugar. People who exercise and lose weight become more insulin sensitive; in other words, the insulin they used to have (or take) is able to do a better job of lowering blood sugar.

For people with Type-II diabetes, it is possible to improve insulin sensitivity <u>permanently</u> by losing weight and keeping it off. This will be discussed in greater detail in chapter 16: "How to Get Off Insulin or Medication (The Weight Loss Factor)".

By exercising and improving insulin sensitivity, many people with Type I diabetes can lower their insulin doses during and after exercise. By exercising and losing weight, many people with Type II diabetes can improve their insulin sensitivity so much that they may be able to stop taking insulin injections or diabetes pills entirely. In fact, it is possible to prevent diabetes through exercise. The more calories a person burns per week exercising, the lower their risk of developing Type-II diabetes!

Edna's good mood wasn't just the result of her better blood sugar control and new excuse for spending money. Exercise produces chemical messengers called "endorphins" that help relieve anxiety and pain, and create a sense of well-being. Endorphins also serve as an appetite suppressant in most people. Exercise really is a wonder drug, but without all the side effects!

What kind of exercise should I do?

The exercise you choose should be based on what you like to do, what you have access to, and what will be safe and reasonable based on your health status and physical abilities. Besides the type of exercise, you should also consider when you will exercise, for how long, how often, and how intensely. Here are some ideas that can help you get started:

WHAT TO DO	• Ideally, low-impact exercises, using large muscle groups rhythmically– such as swimming, biking, walking, rowing, stair climbing, low-impact aerobics, or weight training. • Add "recreational activities" throughout the day such as shopping, yardwork, and extra walking. These help burn extra calories and maintain a high level of insulin sensitivity.
WHEN TO DO IT	• Same time each day for optimal blood sugar control. • After a meal or snack to prevent hypoglycemia and enhance weight loss (Individuals with heart disease should wait 1 hour). • At a time that is usually convenient for you.
HOW OFTEN	• Daily! Think of it as medicine for treating your diabetes. • Aim for 5-7 days per week.
HOW INTENSE	• Moderate. "Fairly Light" to "Somewhat Hard". • Approx. 70% of Maximal Heart Rate – if known. • You should be able to talk comfortably (without getting out of breath) while exercising. However, if you can sing, you may not be exercising hard enough.
HOW LONG	• Aim for 20 to 60 minutes of continuous exercise. The longer you go, the more calories you burn, and the more your blood sugar will drop. • Include a 2-5 minute warm-up & cool-down – a slow, easy version of your exercise activity.
AT WHAT PACE	• Start at a comfortable speed & short duration, such as 10 or 15 minutes at a slow pace. • Build your duration to your goal, such as 30 minutes, before increasing your pace. Once you reach your duration goal, then you can start building on your speed/intensity.

What are the risks of exercise, and how can they be minimized?

The main risks associated with exercise are hypoglycemia (low blood sugar), worsening hyperglycemia (high blood sugar), injuries, and the remote possibility of a heart attack. The good news is that all these risks can be reduced to almost zero by taking a few common sense precautions.

PREVENTING HYPOGLYCEMIA DURING EXERCISE

Low blood sugar is very common in people who take insulin or oral hypoglycemic agents (sulfonylureas - the kind that cause the pancreas to produce extra insulin). Here's why:

When we exercise, the body burns up sugar for energy, and the blood sugar begins to drop. In a person without diabetes, the pancreas starts producing little or no insulin, causing two important things to happen. First, more sugar becomes available for muscles. Second, the adrenaline that we also produce when we exercise goes to the liver and tells it to release its stored-up sugar into the bloodstream. This keeps the blood sugar from going too low. Even a marathon runner will finish a 26-mile run with a normal blood sugar, because his pancreas cuts down insulin production the moment his blood sugar begins to drop.

ADRENALINE

A "stress" hormone that raises blood sugar by releasing the body's sugar stores into the bloodstream. Adrenaline reduces effect of insulin, which takes sugar out of the bloodstream and puts it into the body's cells for energy and storage.

In a person taking insulin or oral hypoglycemic agents, the insulin level in the body does not automatically drop when exercise starts lowering the blood sugar. In fact, it may be very high depending on when and how much insulin or medication was taken.

As a result, the cells keep taking in sugar at a very fast rate. Insulin also "guards" the liver's sugar stores so that adrenaline cannot release it into the bloodstream. The blood sugar continues to drop, and hypoglycemia (low blood sugar) may result.

In a person without diabetes, blood sugar control is on automatic pilot - we don't have to think about it; it just takes care of itself. People who take insulin or oral hypoglycemic agents have to shift into "manual control". Here are a few tips for manually controlling blood sugar during exercise:

- Try to exercise after a meal or snack. Not only will this reduce the likelihood of low blood sugar, but it will also improve your blood sugar control after eating. Drink plenty of fluids prior to exercise, and avoid caffeine - it will make you have to urinate more, and may cause cramps. If you are concerned about getting an upset stomach from exercising after eating, try having just a small amount of fat and protein in your meal.

- Monitor your blood sugar before (and after) exercise to learn how you respond to different activities and when you need to have a snack. Ideally, your blood sugar should be 100 - 180 during exercise. Higher readings may impair your athletic performance, and lower readings put you at risk for low blood sugar. Until you have a chance to learn your blood sugar response to exercise and individual snacking requirements, try using the following as a "starting point":

Pre-Exercise Blood Sugar*	Action To Be Taken
Less than 100	Have 30 grams simple carbohydrate before exercise
100 - 150	Have 15 grams carbohydrate before exercise
150 - 240	No action necessary
Over 240	Check urine for ketones. Do not exercise if ketones are positive

* Note: For optimal blood sugar control, check your sugar one hour prior to exercise, and again just before exercise. If the level is dropping (from, say, 180 to 110), you may need a larger snack than usual.

• Work with your doctor or diabetes educator to reduce your insulin/medication doses.

• Reducing doses that are active during and just after exercise can keep your blood sugar from dropping (see below). However, don't cut your doses too much, or your blood sugar may go very high. As a rule of thumb, start out by reducing your dose of Regular or Humalog by 50%, or if you are adjusting your NPH, Lente or Ultralente, reduce them by 20%. Monitor your blood sugar and make the adjustments accordingly. For example, if you cut your pre-meal regular insulin by 50% and you still get low blood sugar during exercise, try cutting it by 75% next time. Remember, if you have Type-I diabetes, you still need some insulin in your body, so don't eliminate your dose entirely.

If you exercise at this time...	Adjust this insulin.
Pre-Breakfast	NPH, Lente or Ultralente from the night before.
After Breakfast	Pre-breakfast Regular or Humalog.
After Lunch	Morning NPH or Lente, or pre-lunch Regular or Humalog.
Afternoon	Morning NPH or Lente, or pre-lunch Regular
After Dinner	Pre-Dinner Regular or Humalog, and pre-dinner NPH or Lente.

• If exercise is to be performed within an hour after injecting regular or Humalog insulin, inject into a part of your body that won't be very active during exercise, such as the abdomen. Injecting into the leg and then doing leg exercise soon afterward may speed the action of the insulin and lead to low blood sugar.

- During activity lasting more than 90 minutes, check blood sugar at least once per hour and have a snack every 30-60 minutes.

- Since blood sugar may continue to fall for up to 24 hours after strenuous exercise, be prepared to adjust your insulin/medication or eat extra food the following day.

- Highly intense/rigorous activity means that you are burning sugar at a faster rate than during light or moderate exercise. Additional snacking and/or insulin adjustment may be necessary.

Despite taking precautions, low blood sugar can still occur. Always carry a simple sugar source with you (glucose tablets, fruit, sports drink, etc.) and wear medical identification whenever exercising. Treat hypoglycemia immediately and take TIME OUT (15 minutes) for food to be absorbed. Wait until blood sugar is at least 100 before continuing exercise.

TO KEEP A HIGH BLOOD SUGAR FROM GOING HIGHER DURING EXERCISE

High blood sugar can be caused by many different things. Perhaps you ate more than usual. Or perhaps you are under a lot of stress. In either of these cases, exercise will probably not do any harm; it may even bring your blood sugar down and help you to relax.

But what if your blood sugar is high because you are dangerously low on insulin? Your body's cells might be starving for sugar to burn for energy. In this case, high blood sugar might be a sign that your are insulin deficient.

The way to tell if you are deficient in insulin is to check your urine for ketones. A ketone test involves nothing more than urinating on a stick to see if it turns color. If your pre-exercise blood sugar is greater than 240 and you have no clear explanation as to why it is that high, check your urine for ketones. A positive ketone test means that you are deficient in insulin, and exercise will probably make your blood sugar go much higher. Do not exercise if your urine tests positive for ketones.

KETONES

Ketones are dangerous chemicals that are produced when we burn large amounts of fat for fuel. If sugar can't get into our cells (due to insufficient insulin), we are forced to burn only fat for energy, and ketones begin to pollute the bloodstream. If enough ketones build up, it can lead to a life-threatening condition called DKA (diabetic ketoacidosis).

It is also a good idea to delay exercise if your pre-exercise blood sugar is very high. Very high blood sugar can leave you dehydrated and feeling run down. Wait until your blood sugar is under better control before exercising. Also, don't exercise if you have a cold, flu, infection or other acute (short-term) illness. Your body needs all its forces to fight the bug, not the battle of the bulge.

PREVENTING INJURIES

Although some accidents are not predictable or preventable (Guess that's why they call them "accidents"), your chances of suffering common injuries such as muscle strains/soreness, tendon/ligament pulls and sprains, and bone fractures can be reduced significantly by doing the following:

• Warm-up and cool-down by performing a slow version of your exercise activity for 5 minutes at the beginning of your workout.

- Stretch prior to competitive or high impact activities, after warming up. Stretches should be static (no bouncing!) and held for 15-20 seconds, not to a point of pain.

- Start your exercise program at a modest level and progress gradually. Overdoing it at the start is a common cause of soreness and injuries.

- Obtain the proper skills and equipment (including proper footwear) for each type of activity.

- If possible, avoid competitive and high-impact sports. Injuries are much more common when the intensity rises.

PREVENTING SUDDEN HEART ATTACK

Because people with diabetes are at a high risk for silent heart disease, be sure to go over your exercise plan with your doctor before lacing up your sneakers. If you are over age 35, have had diabetes for more than 10 years, or have any additional risk factors such as obesity, high blood pressure, a family history of heart disease, or elevated blood cholesterol/lipids, you should ask your doctor about a stress test before starting to exercise on your own.

Once your doctor has given you the OK you to exercise, you can minimize your risk of heart problems by keeping your exercise intensity moderate and avoiding the tendency to become overly competitive. During aerobic exercises, an adequate warm-up and cool-down help to ensure that your heart can handle the load. Also, remember not to hold your breath when exercising, particularly when lifting weights. Holding your breath while exerting yourself is called a "Valsalva" maneuver, and can place excessive strain on your heart and blood vessels.

Exercise should be stopped if you experience dizziness, shortness of breath, nausea, change in vision, or discomfort in the chest, neck, jaw or arms. Call your doctor immediately if any of these symptoms occur.

OTHER SAFETY ISSUES

1) During exercise, wear clothes that allow your skin to breathe. Rubber or plastic suits are dangerous, and may cause heat stroke or dehydration.

2) Individuals with proliferative retinopathy should limit the intensity of their workouts and avoid activities that cause sudden changes in blood pressure, such as weight lifting and competitive sports.

3) Drink plenty of fluids before, during and after exercise to prevent dehydration and enhance performance. "Sports drinks" which contain small amounts of sodium can enhance re-hydration, but be sure to account for the carbohydrate in these types of drinks.

4) Wear thick cotton socks and comfortable athletic shoes that are appropriate for the activity. Inspect your feet for blisters and sore spots after exercise.

5) After a good workout, stay away from alcohol. Not only does alcohol impair re-hydration; it also masks the symptoms of low blood sugar and may lead to severe hypoglycemia.

How can I keep myself motivated?

As a wise athlete once said, "Exercise is 90% inspiration, and 10% perspiration". The same creativity that went into designing your exercise plan should go into finding ways to make your program fun and rewarding.

Start out by choosing activities you enjoy, and vary your activities from day to day. Make your workouts social by finding a partner, joining a health club, or participating in group activities or leagues. If time is an issue, put your workouts in your appointment book or calendar, and try to catch up on paperwork, phone work or reading while you exercise. To keep yourself entertained, try watching TV (movies or programs on videotape work great!), listening to music, reading or spending time with family or friends.

Remember to set realistic goals for yourself, and reward yourself for meeting your goals. If you like to see results, keep track of your pre/post exercise blood sugar levels, or just observe how your exercise capacity, body shape, weight, measurements and mood improve with each workout!

Key Point
Exercise is like powerful medicine for treating diabetes and preventing complications. Everyone with diabetes should find a way to fit exercise into their diabetes management plan.

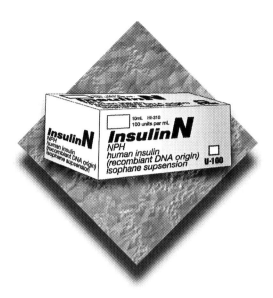

Chapter 6: Insulin

Once upon a time, there was a dreaded disease called diabetes. All who fell victim to this deadly creature suffered a slow and painful death. Granted, people with diabetes could eat all they wanted, but they had lost the ability to turn food into energy. It was like they were continuously filling up their cars, but there was a huge hole in the gas tank. Nobody with diabetes lived very long; most died within a matter of months.

Then one day, two handsome princes named Banting and Best decided to do battle with diabetes. Unlike most monsters which strike at the heart, diabetes attacks the pancreas - the part of the body that makes insulin, a hormone we need to convert food into energy.

Without insulin, you can eat everything in sight, but none of it will do you any good.

Banting and Best said, "Let diabetes do its worst. Who needs the pancreas anyway? If we can get insulin some other way, we can beat the diabetes beast!"

And so, our heroes set out to find a way to replace the insulin that our bodies normally make. They tried all sorts of magical potions until they found just the right mixture - an extract taken from the pancreas of cows and pigs. Trouble was, you couldn't drink this magical potion (it was digested before it ever reached the bloodstream), so it had to be injected with a needle. But given the alternative (a slow and painful death), the needle was preferred by most diabetics surveyed. All of a sudden, they had energy. They felt human. They had life!

Of course, life was still far from normal. Besides the need for daily injections with needles the size of a harpoon, diabetics' blood sugar levels were very poorly controlled. As a result, many died prematurely due to complications such as heart disease and kidney failure. Many also lost their eyesight and required amputations due to poor healing of wounds. The outlook, while not hopeless, was pretty grim.

Today, the magic word (say it, and win a healthy life) is control. Research has shown that the complications of diabetes can be prevented through adequate control of blood sugar levels (see chapter 9: The DCCT Study). Today, people with diabetes can not only live a long life, but a healthy life as well. But don't forget about the basics of diabetes care: everything hinges on insulin.

How Does Insulin Work?

Insulin is the hormone that helps lower blood sugar levels and supply your body's cells with the energy they need. When you eat food, some of the food is broken down to "glucose" - a simple sugar that our cells burn for fuel. The glucose is picked up by the bloodstream and circulated throughout the body. When the pancreas senses that the blood sugar level is rising (just after we eat), it releases insulin into the bloodstream. It also releases a slow, steady stream of insulin all day and night to match the amount of sugar released naturally by the liver.

CELLS

Cells are tiny, living units that make up all the parts of the body. Each cell is separated from the others by a thin membrane. Insulin is required to get sugar through the membrane.

When insulin reaches the body's cells, it opens doors on the surface of the cells to allow the glucose to get inside. Without insulin, the glucose remains in the bloodstream, causing two things to happen:

1) The cells begin to "starve" because they aren't getting enough fuel.

2) The blood sugar level begins to rise very high, clogging up the bloodstream and leading to long-term complications.

In other words, insulin is like the key to your house. By having the key when you need it, you can get into your house to eat, sleep, dress, watch reruns of I Dream of Jeannie, and do whatever it takes to stay healthy and happy. Without the key, you would be locked out - unable to get food, stay warm, and avoid danger. You would be forced to take up residence in the street, which could cause a major traffic jam in front of your house. By getting sugar out of the bloodstream and into your cells, insulin "keys" are critical to your health and survival.

When Are Insulin Injections Necessary?

If the pancreas stops making insulin altogether (Type-I diabetes), your cells would literally starve for fuel. Most people with Type-I diabetes would die within a year without insulin. That is why Type-I diabetes is also called "insulin dependent" diabetes. Everyone with Type-I diabetes must take insulin.

Most people with Type-II diabetes can manage without insulin. Remember, people with Type-II diabetes are usually able to produce some insulin on their own. The problem is often that the insulin is unable to reach the doors on the cells because of too much body fat. In this case, diet, exercise and weight loss may be the only things needed to control the diabetes. If these don't do the trick, certain medications may be prescribed (these will be described in Chapter 8).

Insulin is viewed as a last resort for most people with Type-II diabetes because it has side effects such as weight gain and the tendency to cause low blood sugar. However, if the blood sugar levels are running above normal (70-120 before meals) despite making every attempt to control the diabetes with lifestyle changes and medication, then insulin injections must be started. Otherwise, the risk of complications such as blindness, kidney failure, amputation, nerve damage and heart attack can be very, very high. Insulin may also be needed during times of severe stress, such as illness, surgery, infection, or family crisis.

Since Type-II diabetes is a progressive disease (it tends to become more severe over time), many people wind up on insulin even if they started out doing fine on nothing more than dietary changes and a little bit of exercise. Eventually, one out of three people with Type-II diabetes ends up needing insulin injections.

If you have Type-II diabetes and are told that you should take insulin, don't despair. Celebrate! Soon, you're going to feel much better. Your energy will return, your skin will exude a healthy glow, you won't be running to the bathroom so much, and you will sleep much better. Just remember to stick with your healthy meal plan and exercise, because insulin can cause weight gain if you're not careful.

Where does insulin come from?

In the "old days", insulin was taken from the pancreas of animals such as pigs and cows. This insulin was almost exactly the same as human insulin, but it was different enough to cause problems such as allergic reactions and skin disfigurement in some people. Most insulins available today are exactly the same as the insulin produced by the human pancreas. But don't worry. They don't come from squeezing the pancreas of a human being. They are made in a laboratory using DNA technology, and are referred to as "human insulins". Some are changed slightly to make them act faster or slower, but they rarely cause the kind of side effects that come from using beef and pork insulin.

What are the different types of insulin?

All insulins do the same thing: lower the blood sugar level by getting sugar out of the bloodstream and into the body's cells. However, there are a number of different types of insulin, which vary in terms of how long they take to start working, when they exert their maximum effect, and how long they last once they are injected.

Below is a summary of the main types of insulin:

Insulin Type	Name(s)	Appearance	Starts	Peaks	Stops
Fast Acting	Humalog	Clear	0-15 Min.	30-90 Min.	3-5 Hrs.
Short Acting	Regular	Clear	30-60 Min.	2-4 Hrs.	5-7 Hrs.
Intermediate	NPH*, Lente*	Cloudy	2-4 Hrs.	4-8 Hrs.	12-16 Hrs.
Long Acting	Ultralente*	Cloudy	4-8 Hrs.	8-20 Hrs.	24-36 Hrs.

* Available in beef/pork as well as human insulin version. Beef/pork varieties usually have a longer peak time and duration of action than human insulin.

On the next page is a "graphic" picture showing the action of the different types of insulin:

1. Humalog

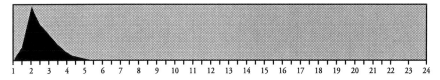

Starts: 0-15 Min.   Peaks: 30-90 Min.   Lasts: 3-5 Hrs.

---

2. Short-Acting Insulin (Regular)

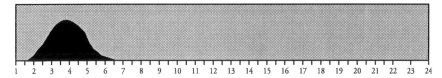

Starts: 1/2-1 Hrs.   Peaks: 2-4 Hrs.   Lasts: 5-7 Hrs.

---

3. Intermediate-Acting Insulin (NPH, Lente)

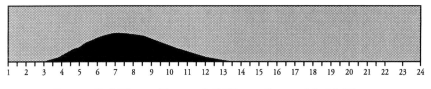

Starts: 2-4 Hrs.   Peaks: 4-8 Hrs.   Lasts: 12-16 Hrs.

---

4. Long-Acting Insulin (Ultra Lente)

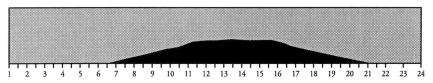

Starts: 4-8 Hrs.   Peaks: 8-20 Hrs.   Lasts: 24-36 Hrs.

73

Some vials of insulin contain a mixture of Regular and NPH insulins. For example, 70/30 insulin contains 70% NPH and 30% Regular insulin. A person taking 20 units of 70/30 is actually taking 14 units of NPH (which peaks in 4-8 hours) and 6 units of regular (which peaks in 2-4 hours).

How Much Does Insulin Lower Blood Sugar?

Insulin works differently in different people. In some people, especially young, thin or active people, a single unit of insulin can lower the blood sugar by more than 100 points. In obese, inactive people, a single unit may lower the blood sugar by just a few points. In general, the more a person weighs, the less each unit of insulin will lower their blood sugar.

UNIT OF INSULN

A single unit insulin, as measured with the markings on a syringe, is equal to 1/100th of a milliliter. A thimble full of insulin would contain about 500 units.

One thing to remember, however, is that all insulins lower blood sugar the same amount; some just take longer to do it than others. All commercially available insulins are U-100, meaning that there are 100 units of insulin in every cc (cubic centimeter). So, if one unit of regular insulin lowers your blood sugar by, say, 30 points, then one unit of Humalog, NPH, Lente or Ultralente will also lower it by 30 points. However, what takes regular insulin 5 hours to accomplish may take NPH or Lente 12 hours; Ultralente 24 hours; and Humalog only 3 hours.

The potency of your insulin will also depend on your blood sugar level at the time the insulin is taken. High blood sugar causes insulin resistance;

insulin doesn't work as well when the blood sugar is high. A unit of insulin may lower your blood sugar by 30 points when your blood sugar is 150, but it may only lower it by 20 points if your blood sugar is 300.

In addition, the action of intermediate (NPH, Lente) and long-acting (Ultralente) insulins can sometimes increase when they are mixed with regular insulin. Many people mix insulins so that one injection will cover the insulin needs for several times of day. For example you can meet your insulin needs at breakfast and lunch by mixing regular insulin (which peaks in the morning) with NPH (which peaks in the afternoon). However, doing so will make the NPH more powerful. If you take 5 units of regular with 18 units of NPH, you get the normal action of 5 units regular, but the 18 units of NPH may act more like 20.

Think Like A Pancreas

The healthy pancreas is like a finely-tuned thermostat in your house. When the temperature begins to fall, the heat turns on just enough to warm the house. Once a comfortable temperature is reached, the thermostat turns the heater off.

To take control of diabetes, you must start to think like a healthy pancreas. Remember, a pancreas normally produces insulin when blood sugar levels rise, so our mission should be to make sure we have just enough working insulin when blood sugar levels are going up — namely after meals and when the liver is releasing extra sugar into the bloodstream (especially during periods of stress and during the pre-dawn hours).

One way we can achieve this is by taking insulin in amounts and at times that mimic what your pancreas would do if it were healthy.

That's why it is so important to know which types of insulin you take and when they are working their hardest. Below is a summary of "insulin actions," based on the peak times of different insulins:

Insulin Type	Time Taken	Period Covered
Humalog	Morning	Breakfast
	Lunchtime	Lunch
	Dinner	Dinner
	Bedtime	Bedtime Snack
Regular	Morning	Breakfast, Mid-Morning
	Lunchtime	Lunch, Early Afternoon
	Dinner	Dinner, Early Evening
	Bedtime	Bedtime Snack, Early Night
NPH/Lente	Morning	Lunch, All Afternoon
	Dinner	Bedtime Snack, All Night
	Bedtime	All Night, Dawn, Pre-Breakfast
Ultralente	Morning	Afternoon, Evening, Nighttime
	Dinner	Nighttime, Morning, Afternoon
	Bedtime	Morning, Afternoon, Evening

Let's look at a few examples to see how the insulin schedule affects blood sugar control.

Dora takes regular and NPH insulin at breakfast and dinner. The morning regular covers her breakfast, the morning NPH covers her lunch, the evening regular covers her dinner, and the evening NPH covers the bedtime snack and nighttime. Her blood sugars average 95 in the morning, 130 at lunch, 210 at dinner, and 115 at bedtime. She reports that she sometimes gets low blood sugar in the middle of the night. What could you suggest to Dora?

One suggestion would be to increase Dora's dose of NPH in the morning. Her blood sugar is going up between lunch and dinner, and since her morning NPH is responsible for this time of day, it would be the logical one to change.

Another suggestion would be to move her evening NPH from dinner to bedtime. That way, the NPH will peak in the morning rather than the middle of the night, and by not mixing the NPH with the regular at dinnertime, the NPH may not be quite as powerful.

<u>Leon</u> takes Ultralente insulin at bedtime. His blood sugars average 200 at breakfast, 150 at lunch, 120 at dinner, and 120 at bedtime. He rarely gets low blood sugar. What suggestions do you have for Leon?

A possible solution would be to take Ultralente twice a day rather than just once. The dose he takes at bedtime doesn't appear to be doing the job during the night. Remember, Ultralente takes several hours to start working, and Leon's liver is releasing sugar into his bloodstream all night long. By taking some Ultralente in the morning and some in the evening, he would have enough insulin working during the night to bring his blood sugar level towards normal.

To prevent high blood sugar as well as low blood sugar, it is important to time your meals and insulin carefully. Thinking like a pancreas means that you should eat just prior to the peak of your insulin. For example, if you take NPH insulin in the morning, it is important to eat about four to six hours later, or you may wind up with low blood sugar. With regular insulin, food should be eaten 30-60 minutes later; with Humalog, food should be eaten right away.

What is the best insulin program?

Whether you would benefit most from several injections a day, pre-mixed insulin or regular vs. Humalog as a fast-acting insulin depends on many factors. It is an important decision that you should make with the help of your doctor. Of course, more injections can be a bit of a nuisance, but they offer better blood sugar control and more flexibility than one or two shots a day. After all, the pancreas gives you insulin many times a day, so why shouldn't you? The key benefits and drawbacks of different insulin programs will be covered in detail in Chapter 13.

Site Rotation

Rotating injection sites is a lot like rotating the tires on your car. It helps to prevent uneven wear and enhances stability.

If you keep injecting insulin into one area of the body for a long time, that area will become hard. The skin will be stiff, and scar tissue will form. The insulin injected into this area will tend to sit for a long time before being released into the bloodstream. As a result, blood sugar levels can be high or inconsistent.

LIPODYSTROPHY

Damage to the fat tissue just below the skin due to repeated injections in the same area. The fat tissue may swell or shrink, causing hard and unsightly areas of skin.

Insulin also absorbs at different rates from different parts of the body. It tends to act fastest when given in the abdomen (stomach), and slowest in the buttocks (behind). The arms and legs can vary depending on the level of physical activity, since exercise speeds absorption of the insulin. Smoking tobacco slows insulin action regardless of the injection site, because it cuts down on blood flow throughout the body.

People who choose their injection sites haphazardly (at random) tend to have unpredictable blood sugar levels because of the different rates of absorption. If you give your morning injection in the abdomen one day and your leg the next day, your insulin will act much more slowly the second day. As a result, your blood sugar may be good one day, high the next.

To prevent skin problems and achieve consistent insulin absorption, the following strategies should be used:

1) For each time of day, use a consistent body part. For example, you might choose to inject your abdomen every morning, leg every evening, and buttocks every night at bedtime. That way, your rates of insulin absorption will be similar from one day to the next, and you won't "wear out" one body part by injecting it too much.

			1	2	3	4
5	6	7	8	9	10	11
11	12	13	14	15	16	17
18	19	20	21	22	23	24
25	26	27	28	29	30	

2) Move the spot of the injection around within each site. If you use your abdomen each day in the morning, try not to use the exact same spot twice in a week. You might imagine that you have a calendar drawn on your stomach, and inject the site that corresponds with

the day of the month. Similar strategies can be used for other body parts as well. Try to space you injections about 1-2 inches apart, and stay away from the belly button, scars, and areas where the skin is becoming hard.

Injecting Insulin

Here are some tips for ensuring proper injection of insulin:

- Syringes come in a variety of sizes, ranging from .25 cc (which hold 25 units) to 1 cc (which hold 100 units). Those taking small doses of insulin would benefit from using the smallest syringe possible because line markings and spaces allow for a more precise dose.

- It is acceptable to re-use syringes up to three or four times. Using a single syringe each day is recommended. Do not attempt to wipe the needle; just re-cap it without touching the tip.

- Alcohol swabs are not necessary. Just make sure the injection site is clean.

- Before drawing up the insulin, make sure it is the type prescribed by your doctor, and mix it by rolling the vial between your palms until it appears to be mixed evenly.

- Inject air into the vial (equal to your dose of insulin) before drawing the insulin into the syringe. Check for and remove air bubbles by pushing the insulin back into the vial and re-drawing the insulin. Never push insulin back into a vial after it has been mixed with another type of insulin.

- When mixing insulins, draw the fast acting (clear) insulin into the syringe before the intermediate or long-acting insulin. This will help to prevent contamination of the vial of fast-acting insulin.

- When mixing Regular and NPH insulin, the mixture may be stored and injected up to three weeks later. Regular can be mixed with Lente, but the injection should be given right away to prevent spoilage of the regular insulin.

- Always double-check your dose before injecting.

- Insulin should be injected into subcutaneous tissue (the fatty layer just below the skin surface). Pinch up an area of skin about two inches wide, insert the needle at a right angle to the skin surface, inject the full dose quickly and remove the syringe before releasing the pinch.

- Dispose of syringes in a safe manner. A thick plastic jug or home sharps container are good for disposing syringes and lancets.

Storing Insulin

It is not necessary to lug around a refrigerator every time you take your insulin with you. Once opened, a vial of insulin is usually good for 30 days when kept at room temperature. It is a good idea to discard the vial after it has been in use for 30 days, even if it is not used up.

It is also a good idea to keep your unopened vials of insulin in the refrigerator until you start using them. This will ensure that they are fresh up until the expiration date marked on the box. NEVER USE INSULIN PAST ITS EXPIRATION DATE.

Also, do not use insulin that appears to have gone bad - if it does not mix evenly, if the color has changed, if "clumps" or "crystals" have formed in the liquid, or if the bottom has a frosty appearance.

Insulin is sensitive to extreme temperatures, so keep it out of direct sunlight, away from heaters, and out of places where it might freeze, such as the coldest part of your refrigerator. And never, ever leave your insulin in your car. Even on a cold day, sunlight can make the inside of your car seem like 100 degrees.

Key Point:
Insulin can save the lives of people with diabetes. But to stay healthy and control blood sugar levels, insulin must be carefully matched to activity and food intake.

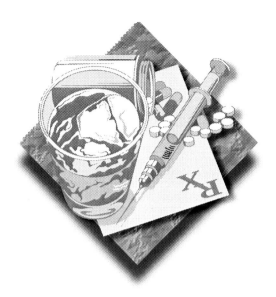

Chapter 7: Insulin Delivery Methods

Yes, my friends, there is more than one way to skin a cat.

It used to be that taking insulin meant jabbing yourself with a needle the size of a harpoon. It was almost an inch long and the width of a fork tine. And after stabbing yourself, you had to boil it for 20 minutes just so you could have the pleasure of using it all over again.

My, how times have changed! Today, there are a number of ways to give yourself insulin in a fast, convenient and virtually pain-free manner. Some of the devices deliver the insulin in a way that achieves better blood sugar control. Some don't even use a needle! Sound interesting? It should be. The insulin delivery method you choose should be based on your own personal needs and preferences. Below is information that you can use to decide which method is best for you: the syringe, the insulin pen, the insulin pump, or the jet injector.

The Syringe

Today's modern syringes are a far less painful imitation of what they used to be. They are lightweight, easy to handle, and disposable. They come in a variety of sizes (25 unit, 30 unit, 50 unit and 100 unit). The benefit of using the smallest syringes possible is that the number markings and spacings are larger, so you can measure your dose more accurately - even in 1/2-unit increments.

Now, let's get down to business. The needle. Needles come in a variety of widths, ranging from 28 gauge to 30 gauge. Here's the tricky part: the larger the gauge, the thinner and more comfortable the needle is.

The length of the needle varies as well. For most adults, the standard 12-13 millimeter needle is optimal. For children and very lean adults, an 8 millimeter needle is available. Remember, the objective is to get the insulin into the subcutaneous tissue (the fatty layer just below the skin), but not so deep that it enters the muscle below the fatty layer. That way, the insulin will be absorbed in a timely and consistent manner.

Most syringe needles are coated with a substance called "silicon" which makes the needle slide in and out of the skin smoothly. With each use, some of the silicon coating wears off, and the tip of the needle becomes slightly less sharp. So, although disposable insulin syringes can be re-used, they are not meant to last forever. Using one syringe a day is usually recommended.

Be sure to dispose of your syringes so that they do not injure you or anyone who handles your trash. Placing them in a plastic, sealed container or sharps disposal is the best way to dispose of your syringes. For information on home sharps containers, contact BD (Becton-Dickinson) or EnviroTech - see Appendix B.

Do NOT attempt to break off the needle before throwing the syringes out. If you are worried about someone taking them out of your trash and using them, simply pull out the plungers and throw them away separately.

Adaptive Devices for Syringe Users

For people with low vision, poor dexterity or anxiety about injecting insulin, a number of special adaptive devices are available. These devices can help ensure that your insulin dose is accurate and easy to inject.

COUNT-A-DOSE (Jordan Medical) is specially designed for those with limited vision who take single or mixed doses of insulin. After attaching the bottles and syringe, the device permits accurate dosing by hearing and feeling "clicks" as each unit is drawn up.

INJECT-EASE (Palco Labs) and INSTAJECT (Jordan Medical) are devices that do the injecting for you. Once the insulin is drawn into the syringe, it is placed inside the device. The device is then placed next to the skin. With the press of a button, the needle is automatically inserted through the skin, ready for you to inject your insulin.

INSULCAP (Diabetic Insulcap) and INSUL-GUIDE (Stat Medical Devices) are small plastic funnels that snap onto the top of the insulin bottle. The shape of the devices helps direct the needle into the center of the rubber stopper on the insulin bottle. It can be very helpful to those who have a hand tremor or poor vision to direct the needle into the bottle when drawing up insulin.

MAGNI-GUIDE (BD) is a magnifier that attaches directly to the syringe. It enlarges the numbers and markings on the syringe so that people with visual impairments can draw up their correct dosage.

Insulin Pens

Insulin pens (Novo Nordisk and BD) are re-usable insulin syringes with insulin cartridges and disposable needles. They offer an easy, accurate, and discreet way to give your insulin anytime, anywhere.

Key Features:
- Plastic or stainless steel casing.
- About the size of a marking pen.
- Disposable insulin cartridges contain approx. 150 units of insulin.
- Disposable needles are available in a variety of lengths & gauges (thickness).
- Dosage is "dialed up" in 1 or 2-unit increments, depending on the device.
- Injection performed with the push of a button.

Key Benefits:
- No need to draw up insulin.
- Makes injections fast and convenient.
- Accurate dosage within 1 or 2 units, depending on the device.
- Discreet - easy to carry and conceal.
- Cuts down on medical waste.

Potential Drawbacks:
- Cannot mix insulins (other than pre-mixed formulations such as 70/30).
- Prefilled pen only offers dosing in 2-unit increments.
- May not be covered by all health insurance policies.

Ideal Candidates:
- People taking multiple injections.
- Those with poor dexterity.
- Students, travelers, and people on the go.
- Those who dine out often.
- Those who feel uncomfortable taking insulin in public places.

Insulin Pumps

An insulin pump (MiniMed, Disetronic) is a beeper-sized device filled with fast-acting insulin. It delivers the insulin to the body through a thin plastic tube called an "infusion set". At the end of the infusion set is either a flexible plastic tube (about 1/2" long) or a small needle that is inserted into the subcutaneous tissue (usually on the abdomen) and taped in place. There it remains for 2-3 days before the infusion set is removed, replaced, and inserted in a new site - much the same way injection sites are rotated.

The pump contains a computer chip that allows the user to program the rate and amount of insulin delivery. Because the pump does not monitor blood sugar levels, it is still up to the user to monitor frequently and tell the pump exactly how much insulin to deliver.

The pump delivers insulin in two different ways: basal insulin and bolus insulin.

Basal insulin is a slow, steady stream of insulin that is designed to match the sugar released by the liver and meet the body's basic metabolic need for energy. Users can program the pump to deliver different basal rates at various times of day to handle routine occurrences such as morning insulin resistance, daytime activity, and the dawn phenomenon.

DAWN PHENOMENON

Before waking up in the morning, the body releases hormones that tend to raise the blood sugar level in "anticipation" of increased energy needs.

Bolus insulin is similar to an insulin injection given to cover a meal or snack. It is usually based on the amount of carbohydrate to be consumed, and must be timed appropriately. The bolus is given in precise amounts prior to each meal or snack by pressing the appropriate buttons on the pump. Together, basal and bolus insulin are the closest thing to a healthy, working pancreas.

Key Features:
- Size and weight similar to a beeper.
- Infusion set tubing comes in a variety of lengths.
- Clip permits secure attachment of pump to belt or waistband.
- Quick-Release mechanism permits temporary detachment for bathing, sports, intimacy.
- Batteries last an average of 2 months.
- Alarms warn of low battery, no insulin delivery.
- Temporary basal rates may be programmed during periods of illness, stress or heavy exercise.

Key Benefits:
- Basal insulin helps stabilize blood sugar levels between meals.
- Reduces the frequency and severity of low blood sugar.
- Permits the user to skip or delay meals.
- Automatic correction of dawn phenomenon.
- Uses only fast-acting insulin for more rapid and predictable absorption.
- User can sleep late without jeopardizing blood sugar control.
- Insulin dosage is very accurate - 1/2 or 1/10-unit increments are possible, depending on the device.
- Insulin may be given anytime, anywhere at the touch of a button.
- Improves blood sugar control during endurance exercise.

Potential Drawbacks:
- Frequent monitoring of blood glucose is essential (4-8 times a day).
- There is a learning curve - control may suffer until use of the pump is mastered.

- Cost of pump and supplies may be prohibitive if insurance does not cover (most insurances DO cover).
- Wearing pump 24-hours a day may be inconvenient.
- There is a risk of ketosis and skin infection.
- Weight gain is possible if the user does not follow an appropriate meal plan.

Ideal Candidates:

- People with Type-I diabetes.
- Those with poor control on injections, frequent low blood sugars, or hypoglycemic unawareness.
- Anyone with an irregular schedule.
- Endurance athletes.
- Women planning or starting pregnancy.
- Children who are very sensitive to small doses of insulin.

Jet Injectors

Jet Injectors (Health Mor, Medi-Ject) are needle-free, spring-loaded devices that spray a stream of insulin through the skin. They offer a variety of pressure settings to help ensure that the insulin penetrates the skin but does not go so deep as to cause pain or bruising.

To use a jet injector, a plastic adapter is first attached to the vials of insulin. The adapters permit the insulin to be drawn into the device's chamber by dialing up the appropriate dose in single or half-unit increments. The vial of insulin is then removed, and the injection pressure (depth) is set. The device is placed against the skin, and the insulin is infused with the touch of a button.

It is important to note that insulin given with a jet injector tends to start working sooner, peak faster, and stop working earlier than insulin given with a syringe. This is due to the "spray-like" dispersion that a jet injector creates.

Key Features:

- Hand-held device about the size of a large marking pen.
- Mixing insulins is possible.
- Multiple pressure settings for different skin types and body parts.
- Visual readout and "clicks" permit accurate dosing within 1/2 unit.
- No batteries. Device is spring-operated.

Key Benefits:

- Needle-free means minimal discomfort, discreet injections, and safety.
- Enhanced insulin absorption improves after-meal blood sugar control.
- Easy on skin; does not cause tissue damage.
- Cuts down significantly on medical waste.
- Delivers dosage accurately within 1/2 unit.

Potential Drawbacks:

- Bruising, pain or inaccurate dose if injection is not performed properly.
- May not be covered by some health insurances.
- Takes longer to perform an injection.
- Requires weekly cleaning.
- Rapid absorption may limit duration of intermediate and long-acting insulin.

Ideal Candidates:

- Anyone who takes insulin.
- Children age five and up.
- Older adults who are anxious about using needles.

- Visually impaired persons.
- Those with above-target blood sugar levels after meals.
- Those who are reluctant to draw-up insulin in public places.

On the Horizon

Current research is exploring more convenient and effective ways to deliver insulin. For example, companies are examining "nasal insulin" - an insulin spray that is absorbed through the nasal passages. Others are testing an "insulin patch" - a device that releases insulin through the skin in a time-release manner.

Finally, "insulin pills" are still being developed. These pills would protect insulin from the acids and enzymes of the digestive tract long enough for the insulin to be absorbed into the bloodstream. Watch your newspapers and diabetes journals for more information on these devices as they become available.

> **Key Point:**
> Today's syringes and insulin delivery devices offer safe, comfortable and effective ways to give insulin. Discuss these devices with your doctor and take advantage of the benefits they have to offer.

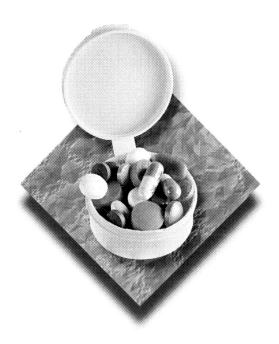

Chapter 8: Oral Medications

Ever since the discovery of insulin in the early part of the century, scientists have tried to find a way to put insulin into pill form. So far, their attempts have been unsuccessful because insulin taken by mouth is digested before it can reach the bloodstream. However, for people with Type-II diabetes, there are many different kinds of pills that can improve blood sugar control via "indirect" methods, such as reducing the liver's release of sugar, slowing the absorption of sugar from the digestive tract, helping make the body's cells more sensitive to the insulin produced by the pancreas, and increasing the amount that it can produce.

Although the diabetes pills developed recently have fewer side effects than those from years past, all diabetes pills carry certain risks that must be weighed against their benefits. It is up to <u>you</u> to learn about the latest advances in diabetes medications and find out which ones can benefit you the most.

Who Needs Diabetes Pills?

Diabetes pills are meant for people with Type-II diabetes who are unable to control their diabetes through healthy meal planning, exercise and weight loss. Remember, a healthy lifestyle is your first and most important line of defense against Type-II diabetes. Pills do not take the place of healthy living, nor should they be used without trying lifestyle changes first. However, not everyone achieves better blood sugar control with weight loss. And even in those who do, the pancreas may start to wear down over time. For these reasons, about half of all people with Type-II diabetes wind up taking diabetes pills.

Sulfonylureas: Oral Hypoglycemic Agents

Sulfonylureas, also called Oral Hypoglycemic Agents (or OHAs, for short) were first developed in the 1950s. These drugs make the pancreas produce larger amounts of insulin and make the muscles, liver and other tissues of the body slightly more sensitive to insulin. THESE PILLS ARE NOT INSULIN. They just help the body make more insulin, and help it to work a little bit better. If the pancreas is unable to make any insulin at all, OHAs will not do any good; it would be like beating a dead horse.

OHAs work best in people who have had diabetes for less than 10 years and are not severely obese. They should not be used during pregnancy, or by those who have liver or kidney disease or an allergy to sulfa.

Just like cars, OHAs have different models. The older models are referred to as "first generation" OHAs. These include:

- Chlorpropamide (brand name Diabinese)
- Tolazamide (Tolinase)
- Tolbutamide (Orinase)
- Acetohexamide (Dymelor)

Just like first-year cars, first-generation OHAs will do the job, but they have their share of problems. For starters, they tend to hang around for a very long time (up to 36 hours), and may cause water retention and loss of sodium. They also interact with many over-the-counter drugs, including aspirin. Most importantly, first generation OHAs have a tendency to cause low blood sugar and weight gain by stimulating the pancreas to produce too much insulin.

"Second Generation" OHAs are more potent and have fewer "bugs" than the first-generation drugs. However, they can still cause low blood sugar and weight gain.

Second generation OHAs include:

- Glyburide (brand names Diabeta, Micronase). These are long-acting and are good for lowering fasting (morning) blood sugar levels.
- Glipizide (Glucotrol, Glucotrol XL): This is short acting and is good for lowering blood sugar after meals. Glucotrol XL is longer acting and also helps lower fasting blood sugar.
- Glybenclamide (Glynase): Similar to Glyburide.
- Glimeperide (Amaryl): This is long-acting; it works primarily by making the body's cells more sensitive to insulin and by stimulating the pancreas to produce more insulin.

It should be noted that OHAs tend to lose their effectiveness over time, especially if the person taking them gains weight or does not comply with other aspects of their diabetes management program such as proper meal planning or exercise.

In addition, medical problems that call for the use of steroids (such as Prednisone), estrogen or beta blockers will reduce the effectiveness of OHAs.

If you are currently taking an OHA for your diabetes and your fasting blood sugar readings are above 150, it may be time to discuss another form of therapy with your doctor. On the flip side, if you are taking OHAs and experience low blood sugar several times a week, it may be time to talk to your doctor about reducing your dosage or eliminating the pills entirely!

Combined Therapy

As mentioned earlier, OHAs tend to lose their effectiveness over time because the pancreas tends to wear out and lose its ability to produce insulin. If you have "maxed out on oral agents", it means that you are taking the largest possible dose of OHA and your blood sugar is still not coming down to the normal range. You are probably tired a lot and don't have much energy. Odds are you are going to the bathroom often and haven't had a full night's sleep in quite some time. Your weight may even be up a bit from when you first started on the OHA.

Time for some fresh blood. Insulin to the rescue! A single dose of insulin at night, taken in conjunction with a reduced dose of OHA, may be just the ticket. Taking NPH or Lente (intermediate-acting insulin) at bedtime will help lower your blood sugar through the night and bring your fasting readings under control. It will allow you to sleep through the night and feel more energetic the next morning. And by starting the day with a good blood sugar level, you stand a much better chance of keeping it under control the rest of the day.

Remember, Type II diabetes is a progressive disease. As time goes on, your pancreas is likely to produce less and less insulin. At some point, OHAs may be useless because the pancreas cannot produce any additional insulin. Your blood sugar levels during the day (lunch, dinner and bedtime) may become elevated, and additional insulin injections may be necessary. However, as long as OHAs are still doing the job at keeping your blood sugar levels under control, it is best to use them and minimize the amount of insulin you are taking. This will ultimately reduce your chances for complications such as high blood pressure, heart disease and stroke.

Metformin: The Risk Reducer

Recently approved for use in the United States is a new drug for improving blood sugar control: METFORMIN. It has been used safely in Canada and Europe for many years in people with diabetes who do not have kidney or liver disease.

Metformin (Glucophage) works differently than OHAs in that it does not force the pancreas to produce more insulin. As a result, Metformin does not result in low blood sugar. It also does not cause weight gain the way OHAs can.

Here is how Metformin works:

1. First and foremost, Metformin makes the liver and muscles more sensitive to insulin. By doing so, it keeps the liver from releasing too much sugar into the bloodstream, and helps the muscle cells take sufficient amounts of sugar out of the bloodstream. The result is lower blood sugar levels in the morning, and better blood sugar control after meals.

2. By making the body much more sensitive to insulin, the pancreas can cut down on its insulin production. Not only does this help to "rest" the pancreas — it also has beneficial side effects such as lowering triglyceride levels (fats in the blood), blood pressure and appetite.

If you are already taking insulin or OHAs, Metformin may allow them to work much better. Remember the saying, "the whole is greater than the sum of the parts." In other words, the effect of taking Metformin and OHAs together is greater than if you took each one individually. An OHA alone may lower your blood sugar by 30 points, and Metformin alone may lower it by 30. But together, they might lower your blood sugar by 100 points rather than 60. The same goes for Metformin and insulin. Metformin "amplifies" the effects of insulin and OHAs several times.

There are a few possible side effects associated with Metformin. In some patients, it can cause bloating, indigestion and diarrhea. And since the drug is eliminated from the body by the kidneys, it should not be used by anyone who has kidney disease. It should also not be used during pregnancy. People taking Metformin are warned against drinking any alcohol, as this may lead to serious complications.

Metformin is a "risks reducer" because it has so many health benefits besides the obvious lowering of blood sugar levels. However, as with OHAs, Metformin will only help if you continue to keep a healthy diet and exercise regularly.

Precose: For High Blood Sugar After Meals

It's 8 o'clock at night, and you are starving. You head for the fridge, but before you have a chance to open the door, a number is staring you in the face. No, it's not the number of overeaters anonymous or your local diabetes support group. It is the number for the Pizza Delivery Guy just up the road.

30 minutes later, he arrives, bearing cheese-laden gifts that would bring a smile to even the wealthiest of kings. You tip him mightily, turn on the tube, and enjoy the ultimate of eating frenzies.

No matter that two hours later your blood sugar is running somewhere between 300 and 400. After all, you see your doctor every three months, and when he checks your pre-breakfast fasting blood sugar, it's always pretty good.

What you might be forgetting is that, to your body, blood sugar after meals is every bit as important as blood sugar before meals. The DCCT (Diabetes Control and Complications Trial) proved that tight blood sugar control throughout the day and night is important for preventing long-term complications of diabetes. Blood sugar levels before meals are typically the lowest readings of the day, because blood sugar rises after we eat. A 100 before a meal can easily become 180 after the meal. 150 can become 250. And 200... well, you don't want to know.

There are a number of ways to lower blood sugar levels after a meal, such as including fiber in the meal, using fast-acting insulins and medications, and exercising soon after eating. These will be discussed in detail in Chapter 13: Intensifying Control.

Now, there is one more weapon in your arsenal. Precose is a new pill that brings down blood sugar levels after meals. It does this by *slowing down* the digestion of carbohydrates, and slowing the release of sugar into the bloodstream.

Let's take that Pizza as an example. First, Precose slows down the digestion of the crust (which is mostly carbohydrate), so blood sugar is slower to rise. Precose also makes it tough for the sugar to reach the bloodstream, sort of like building a wall it must climb over. As a result, rather than having the sugar hit your bloodstream all at once, it rises very slowly and gradually, allowing your pancreas to make enough insulin to keep it from going very high.

On average, Precose helps lower blood sugar levels after meals by 50 points. Precose has very few side effects, but it should not be used in people who have kidney disease or chronic intestinal problems such as ulcerative colitis or Crohn's disease. Also, if you already take insulin or OHAs and add Precose to your program, be aware that certain foods may not be appropriate for treating low blood sugar. Since Precose slows the digestion of complex starches, only simple sugars should be used in the treatment of hypoglycemia.

Drug Type	Methods of Action	Major Side Effects
Sulfonylureas (OHAs)	• Increases Insulin Production • Improves Insulin Sensitivity	• Hypoglycemia • Weight Gain
Metformin	• Blocks Sugar Release From the Liver • Increases Insulin Sensitivity Throughout the Body	• Intestinal Upset
Precose	• Slows Digestion of Carbohydrates • Slows Absorption of Sugar Into the Blood Stream	• Intestinal Upset

Key Point:

There are a number of pills that can be used to improve blood sugar control in Type II diabetes. But don't forget that pills are not the "cure". Diabetes management still requires that you follow a sensible meal plan and exercise regularly.

Section III:

Day-to-Day Control

Tony is a nut when it comes to home repairs. His garage is chock full of every conceivable kind of repair gadget and power tool known to modern man. He has spent a fortune and invested a considerable amount of time putting together the finest workshop in town, but there is one problem: Tony hasn't the faintest idea of how to use all the stuff. So despite having an entire hardware store in the garage, Tony's house is falling apart.

In section II, we presented the tools of diabetes management: meal planning, exercise, diabetes pills, insulin and insulin delivery devices. But as Tony has demonstrated to a "T", good tools are useless without the knowledge and skills to use them effectively.

This section focuses on the day-to-day management of blood sugar levels. We will explore the role of blood sugar monitoring and how to use the results to fine-tune your control. Some of the most common sources of blood sugar variations will also be presented so that you can start eliminating trouble makers and take control of your diabetes. You will learn how to utilize your diabetes management tools to improve your blood sugar control and why it is to your advantage to do so. Finally, strategies for dealing with illness and low blood sugar will be spelled out in terms that are easy-to-understand and apply.

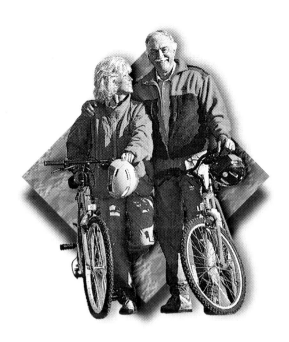

Chapter 9: The DCCT Study: What It Means For <u>You</u>

Around the turn of the century, just after the discovery of insulin, Dr. Elliot Joslin was convinced that just giving insulin wasn't good enough. After all, insulin could extend the lives of people with diabetes for many years, but the complications of diabetes (blindness, heart disease, kidney failure, amputation, nerve disorders) made life difficult and in some cases unbearable.

Dr. Joslin believed that people deserve more than life. They deserve quality life. He believed that many of the complications of diabetes could be prevented or delayed by keeping blood sugar levels as close to normal as possible. For years, doctors fed this advice to their patients, but without much conviction or support. After all, there was no hard evidence to support the belief that tight control of blood sugar lowers the risk of complications.

The "Show Me" State

As they say in Missouri, "Show Me, Don't Tell Me." Without any real proof of the value of tight blood sugar control, doctors and patients should be skeptical of intensive diabetes management. Tight control of blood sugar takes more work, costs more, and carries a greater risk of low blood sugar than "loose" control. And to top it off, many people with tight control still suffer from the long-term complications of diabetes.

One doctor said it best when he said, "Why should I ask my patients to take more shots, monitor more often, and experience more episodes of hypoglycemia if it may not do them any good in the end?" Indeed, people deserve to know if tight control makes a difference, or if it is just a ploy to help the test strip manufacturers make more money.

Along Comes the DCCT

In the early 1980s, an "All-Star Team" of prominent diabetes doctors and researchers gathered at the National Institutes of Health (NIH) to figure out a way to answer the question, "Does tight control of blood sugar help prevent diabetic complications?"

They decided to conduct a nationwide research project called the Diabetes Control and Complications Trial (DCCT). The study involved more than 1400 people with Type I diabetes in 25 cities in the United States and Canada. Because it can take many years for complications to develop, the study took almost 10 years to complete.

Half of the group (the <u>intensive treatment group</u>) was treated with multiple injections of insulin (3 or more shots a day, or use of an insulin pump), and monitored their own blood sugars four or more times each day. The insulin doses were adjusted based on food intake, exercise and blood sugar test results. For example, a participant might increase their morning insulin if their blood sugar was 200, or reduce it if morning exercise was planned. The goal was to keep pre-meal blood sugars as close as possible to a target range of 80-140.

The intensive treatment group received a hospital stay at the beginning of treatment, followed by weekly to monthly visits with the clinical team. Each participant also received a complete diet and exercise plan.

So, what about the other half of those 1400 participants? They simply followed the diabetes management regimen that was being used by most people at the time the study was started. This included one or two shots of insulin a day, daily blood sugar checks (usually first thing in the morning), and visits to the doctor's office every three months. Participants in this group, called the <u>conventional treatment group</u>, were not instructed on how to make adjustments to their insulin doses. They also received basic diet and exercise information rather than individualized plans.

Throughout the study, participants were screened and tested for diabetes complications, particularly retinopathy (diabetic eye disease), neuropathy (nerve disease), nephropathy (kidney disease) and blockages within large blood vessels (macrovascular disease) - the type that might lead to amputation, stroke or heart attack

To evaluate each participant's overall blood sugar control, a test called a Glycosylated Hemoglobin was performed every three months. This blood test provides an indication of the "average" blood sugar for the previous two to three months, and will be discussed in greater detail in chapter 11.

What were the results?

Not surprisingly, the conventional treatment group had blood sugars that were well above normal throughout the study. The glycosylated hemoglobin for the group averaged 8.9, which indicated average blood sugars of approximately 210.

The intensive treatment group also had blood sugars that were above normal, but not nearly as much as the conventional group. The intensive group had an average glycosylated hemoglobin of 7.2, which indicated average blood sugars of about 155.

But here is the important finding: TIGHTER BLOOD SUGAR CONTROL DECREASED THE INCIDENCE OF COMPLICATIONS SIGNIFICANTLY. Putting it in plain English, the people in the intensive treatment group developed fewer complications than people using conventional treatment. They experienced 76% less eye disease, 56% less kidney disease, and 60% less nerve disease (see below):

Average Blood Sugar

Conventional Treatment: 210
Intensive Treatment: 155

Progression of Nephropathy (Kidney Disease)

Conventional Treatment / Intensive Treatment

Development of Retinopathy (Eye Disease)

Conventional Treatment / Intensive Treatment

Risk of Neuropathy (Nerve Damage)

Conventional Treatment / Intensive Treatment

For those who already had complications prior to the study, intensive treatment helped to slow down the progression of the complications dramatically. This meant that people with mild retinopathy kept their vision for much longer. Those whose kidney function was already impaired were able to go for much longer before needing dialysis or a transplant. And those with impaired nerve sensation did not appear to get worse very quickly.

As far as the macrovascular, or large blood vessel complications (heart attack, stroke, amputation), it should be noted that the participants in the study were relatively young (average age was 27) and healthy, other than having Type I diabetes. Even though the intensive treatment group had fewer macrovascular complications, there were so few cases of heart attack, stroke and amputation that it could not be proven statistically that intensive management makes a difference. However, experts believe that if the study had lasted longer, there would have been sufficient evidence to prove that intensive control lowers the risk of large blood vessel disease. So, the bottom line is that CONTROL MATTERS. The better you control your blood sugar, the lower your risk of long-term complications. Does this guarantee that you won't get complications? Of course not. But it does improve your odds considerably.

How low should my blood sugar be?

Remember, even the intensive therapy group did not achieve "normal" blood sugar levels all the time. Perhaps the best news to come out of the DCCT study is that you don't need to have perfect blood sugars to reduce your risk of complications. In fact, any improvement that you can make will lower your risk (see next page):

Risk of Complications

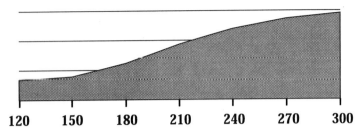

| 120 | 150 | 180 | 210 | 240 | 270 | 300 |

In other words, if your average blood sugar is 300, you don't need to get it down to 150 right away. Lowering it to 250 will reduce your risk of complications a little bit. If you are 250 now, getting it down to 200 or 175 will help. When it comes to reducing your risk of complications, every little bit helps. And it doesn't matter what kind of diabetes you have, whether you use insulin or pills, or even if you control your diabetes through a steady diet of sushi and beach volleyball. Better control means a lower risk of diabetic complications for everyone with diabetes. (For helpful hints on intensifying your blood sugar control, see Chapter 13).

Overcoming the Obstacles to Intensive Control

As our kids keep reminding us, nothing in life is free. There are prices to pay for intensive diabetes control, but there are also ways to minimize the costs. And it is better to be penny wise than dollar foolish: A small investment today can reap tremendous benefits (avoidance of complications) down the road.

One possible cost is the risk of low blood sugar (hypoglycemia). Low blood sugar was three times more common in the intensive treatment group than in the conventional group, simply because there was less margin for error. A 100 point drop in blood sugar (due to exercise or a delayed meal, for example) would probably produce hypoglycemia in the intensive group, but probably would not drive the sugar down enough to be too low in the conventional group. There is also a tendency to lose the warning signs of low blood sugar (shaking, sweating, rapid heart beat) when hypoglycemia occurs often.

The good news is that you can reduce your risk of hypoglycemia by making a few common-sense adjustments to your insulin doses and food intake. Strategies for preventing hypoglycemia will be presented in Chapter 14.

Weight gain is another potential problem. While the average weight gain was only a few pounds for people in the intensive treatment group, it is important to consider why weight gain occurs. In the conventional treatment group, blood sugar was usually over 200, while the intensive group averaged about 150. Whenever blood sugar is over 180, the kidneys start to eliminate some of the sugar through the urine. That means that people in the conventional group were hitting the bathroom an awful lot to urinate. The intensive treatment group did not urinate away as much sugar as the conventional group. In other words, both groups probably ate the same number of calories, but the intensive group did a better job of retaining what they ate. Many of the calories consumed by the conventional group wound up being flushed away.

One other downside of intensive management is the cost. The average cost per year for supplies, prescriptions, medical care, etc. is about $1500 to $2000 for conventional treatment, versus $3000 to $4000 for intensive treatment. Some insurance companies are realizing the value of this investment, however, since the cost of laser treatment of the eyes, kidney dialysis or heart bypass is typically in the tens or hundreds of thousands of dollars.

If your insurance does not cover the cost of your supplies and treatment, ask yourself this: Is it worth a thousand dollars to be able to see, or to have working kidneys rather than needing ongoing dialysis treatments, or to keep from losing your feet?

Good blood sugar control takes work, but it is well worth the effort. It is up to you to demand the best from your health care providers, just like a quarterback leads a football team. To be a leader, you have to take on responsibility and see it through. Go for the touchdown - go for better control of your diabetes!

Key Point:

Any improvement you can make in your blood sugar control will lower your risk of diabetes complications.

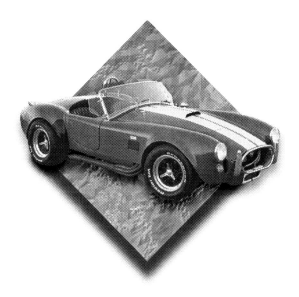

Chapter 10: Blood Glucose Monitoring

Imagine, if you will, that you are behind the wheel of an expensive sports car - one that you have saved for your entire life. You find yourself mesmerized by the smell and feel of the rich leather seats, the hum of the powerful engine, the serenity of the tinted glass, and the jet-like display of controls in the dashboard. You tool down a popular drag in the heart of downtown, heads turning as you motor by. You suddenly realize that you have lost touch with everything that is going on. You can't see, you can't hear, you can't feel or smell or, well, <u>anything</u>. The car is speeding out of control, and you struggle helplessly to avoid an accident. But without your senses to guide you, your chances are somewhere between slim and none.

Trying to manage your diabetes without checking your blood sugar is like driving a car without having any of your senses. You might coast along for a little while, but sooner or later you're bound to crash and burn.

Self-monitoring of blood glucose (SMBG) has brought diabetes care from the doctor's office to your fingertips (literally!). Gone are the days when the doctor checks your blood every 2-3 months and tells you everything is fine, or decides to change your medication based on one reading. Some people do everything they can to get their blood sugar into a good range just in time for their visit to the doctor. Some exercise just before coming in; some change their diet radically; some even fast beforehand. What they don't realize is that today's best doctors don't base their patients' control on one lone test result - and neither should you.

What you can get out of monitoring

Just the other day, a patient came into the office and asked if we had any glucose tablets because she felt like she had low blood sugar. We checked her blood sugar and found that it was 280. Besides saving her from driving her blood sugar even higher, checking her blood proved an important point: IT IS ALMOST IMPOSSIBLE TO PREDICT YOUR BLOOD SUGAR BY THE WAY YOU FEEL.

You can feel pretty good with blood sugars that are in the 150-200 range, but this would be putting you at an increased risk for complications. You can also feel like you have low blood sugar when it is actually high. Likewise, many people do not experience the usual symptoms of low blood sugar (shaking, sweating, rapid heartbeat) until the blood sugar drops dangerously low. In other words, the way you feel is not a good way to estimate your blood sugar level. You need to check your blood.

Checking your blood sugar is not without its rewards. Sure, there is some time, expense and discomfort involved, but look at all you can get out of it:

1. Checking your blood sugar before meals can allow you to adjust your insulin or medication doses appropriately. Let's say your blood sugar is 250 prior to breakfast. Rather than taking your normal dose of insulin, you can increase your dose so that you won't have high blood sugar all day long. Consistently high (or low) readings at a certain time of day should tell you that an adjustment needs to be made to your meal plan, exercise schedule, or insulin/medication. This will be discussed in greater detail in Chapter 13: Intensifying Control and Making Adjustments.

2. Checking your blood sugar after meals can teach you how different foods affect your blood sugar. Some foods may cause a rapid rise, while others are slow to hit your bloodstream. You may find that certain food combinations cause more or less of a rise than you expected. For example, many people find that their blood sugar goes higher when they eat out than when they dine at home. Others find that meals rich in fiber cause less of a blood sugar rise after the meal than meals that are low in fiber. It is only through monitoring that you can learn the impact of foods, and more importantly, how to make adjustments for them.

3. If you are trying to lose weight by cutting back on your calories, you will see improvements in your blood sugar levels long before you see noticeable changes in your weight. Not only is this motivational, but it also shows that your efforts are working to control your diabetes.

4. If you are losing weight, monitoring will tell you if it is due to loss of sugar through the urine (and breakdown of body tissues due to insufficient insulin), or genuine weight reduction that comes from burning more calories than you take in. Any time your blood sugar

exceeds the renal threshold, your kidneys will start eliminating sugar through the urine. Many of the calories you are taking in will wind up being urinated away rather than being put into your body's cells for energy. You can easily lose several hundred calories a day through the urine. As a result, you could be losing a great deal of weight. However, this can be very unsafe since it can lead to dehydration as well as breakdown of important body components such as muscle. If you find that you are losing weight due to high blood sugar, talk to your doctor about changing your insulin or medication dosage.

RENAL THRESHOLD

This is the point at which the kidneys start putting sugar into the urine. In most people, sugar starts leaking into the urine when the blood sugar is above 180.

---

5. Monitoring can help you improve athletic performance and prevent low blood sugar during exercise. Checking your blood before exercise can tell you if you need a snack or more insulin; optimal performance takes place when the blood sugar is between 80 and 180. Checking your blood during and after exercise can help you determine the best adjustments to insulin/medication doses, as well as the optimal amount and frequency of snacks. Seeing how much your blood sugar comes down when you exercise can also provide a sense of accomplishment and inspiration.

6. During illness, the body's insulin needs can go way up. Before we have a chance to adjust insulin doses, the blood sugar can go up as well. By checking the blood sugar every 4-6 hours, you can determine whether your insulin doses are appropriate, or if you need a "booster" dose of fast-acting insulin prior to meals. (See chapter 15: Dealing with High Blood Sugar, Illness and Infection)

7. As mentioned earlier, it is possible to have symptoms of low blood sugar without actually having low blood sugar. When the blood sugar is very high - in the 200s, 300s or 400s - you may feel shaky, weak and hungry. When the blood sugar falls rapidly, from say 250 to 150 in less than an hour, you may experience low blood sugar-like symptoms as well. Of course, treating a low blood sugar with fast-acting carbohydrates in these situations will only make your control worse. It is best to check your blood before treating what seems like a low blood sugar. If you feel unusually hungry, it is also a good time to check since high blood sugar can cause excessive hunger.

8. If your blood sugar is tightly controlled, you may lose some of the early warning signs of low blood sugar. These symptoms, which include shaking, sweating, and heart palpitations, occur when the blood sugar is near or just below 70. However, if you no longer get these early symptoms, the blood sugar may drop dangerously low before any symptoms are detected. Frequent monitoring of blood sugar levels can help you to catch low blood sugar before it gets to be a serious problem.

9. One of the extra benefits of frequent blood sugar monitoring is that it may help you to catch an illness, infection or stressful situation early on. When your readings suddenly go up and stay high, there is a strong possibility that you are experiencing a great deal of stress, and the high blood sugars are telling you that you had better find a relief valve (such as exercise, relaxation, or a new way of perceiving things). Or perhaps the high readings are due to an infection. Catching an infection early makes it easier to treat and can prevent it from spreading. Finally, high blood sugar may be an indication that you are not receiving an adequate dose of insulin. Perhaps your insulin vial has gone bad, or the insulin is not absorbing well from the site where it was injected. There may be a problem with your injection technique. Or perhaps your dosage is just too low to meet your body's needs. In

any case, insufficient insulin means that your body's cells are being deprived of the sugar they need to burn for energy. Over time, this can lead to the breakdown of body tissues, and a life-threatening condition called ketoacidosis. Once again, catching the problem early can help you regain control and quite possibly save your life.

What is the best way to test?

Sometimes, technology can be a real pain in the neck. Hot air dryers in restrooms, for example. But sometimes, technology produces things that are really helpful, like blood glucose meters.

Today, blood glucose meters are fast, easy to use, and accurate. It used to take a nurse with a large needle and a complete laboratory to do a blood sugar analysis. Now, a simple prick of the finger and a device the size of a pocket calculator can do the trick in less than a minute.

Of course, there are many different types of meters and manufacturers (Bayer, Boehringer Mannheim, Cascade Medical, Home Diagnostics, LifeScan, Medisense - see Appendix B), all of whom will tell you that their machine is the best. Since your meter is going to get a lot of use... heck, it's going to be like your best buddy... it makes sense to do some comparison shopping before settling on a particular meter.

Some meters have a built-in memory that keeps track of your blood sugar readings along with the date and time. Some even allow you to enter your insulin doses and "event markers" for later analysis. There are a number of computer programs that will allow you to download the data from your meter and perform basic data analysis, complete with graphs and charts. (See appendix B - MediLife's Balance PC, MediSense's Precision Link, Boehringer Mannheim's Accu-Chek PDM Pro, LifeScan's In Touch, HealthWare's Level)

The size of meters varies from the size of a videocassette to a credit card to a fountain pen. Some have big buttons for easy handling; some have no buttons at all. The time it takes a meter to read a result can vary from a few seconds up to one minute, so if you plan to do a lot of checking, look for one that works fast. Some require periodic cleaning, while others need no cleaning at all. The power source can vary as well. Some have built-in batteries that last for the life of the meter, while others have batteries that need to be replaced every so often. For the visually impaired, some offer large readout or a voice synthesizer (Home Diagnostics, Lighthouse - see Appendix B).

The one thing that all meters have in common is the need to place a drop of blood on a test strip. This is the feature that can make or break a meter, because if the test strip is difficult to dose properly, the meter can produce false readings. Look for a meter whose test strips have a small, rounded test area rather than a large or square-shaped test area (see below):

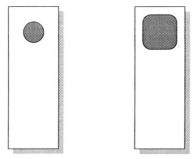

Easier to Dose   Harder to Dose

Most meters work by electronically measuring the color change on the test strips. There are chemicals in the test strips that change color when mixed with sugar. The more sugar, the greater the color change. Some meters will shoot a tiny pulse of electricity through the blood sample. The more sugar the blood contains, the faster the impulse travels.

What about urine testing?

Diabetes mellitus, by definition, means "sweet urine". Back in ancient Egypt, medicine men used to taste the urine to see if it contained sugar (sweet urine meant diabetes and imminent death for the victim).

Today, urine testing for sugar is as obsolete as applying leeches. Urine testing used to be popular before home blood glucose testing became readily available. Because we tend to spill sugar into the urine when the blood sugar level is above 180, higher blood sugar can be detected by testing the urine for sugar.

But there are many problems with urine testing. First of all, it will only tell you when the blood sugar is high. It will tell you nothing if the blood sugar is under 180. There is a lag time of 1-2 hours between the time when the blood sugar is high and when sugar appears in the urine. Your blood sugar could have just risen to 250, but your urine could contain no sugar because it hasn't had time to spill over into the urine. Or, your blood sugar could be 50 and you could have sugar in your urine from a high level earlier in the day. Therefore, testing glucose in the urine is neither accurate nor reliable. If you are still testing your urine for sugar, get yourself a meter and start testing your blood.

Testing Tips

By using proper technique when checking your blood sugar, you can minimize the pain and cost, and ensure the accuracy of your blood sugar readings.

When pricking your finger, it is best to use a lancing device. Some lancing devices (Boehringer Mannheim's Softclix, Palco Labs' Auto-Lancet, BD's Lancet Device, Stat Medical's Quik-Let) have caps with different thicknesses that allow you to adjust the depth of the lancet.

With few exceptions, most lancing devices can use the same lancets. Many people find Ultra Fine lancets (B-D) to be among the best because they have a thinner point than most other lancets.

Always start with the thickest cap on your lancing device (this produces the shallowest finger prick). If this does not produce enough blood, go to a thinner cap. Achieving the proper depth (not too deep, not too shallow) will help to eliminate unnecessary pain and make sure you get a good drop of blood every time. And this will keep you from wasting test strips.

It is best to use several different fingers for testing your blood - especially the 3rd, 4th and 5th fingers on each hand (avoid the index finger and thumb). Rather than pricking the very tip of the finger (this is where most of the sensitive nerve endings are), try pricking toward the sides. It is not necessary to wipe your fingers with alcohol, but washing your hands with warm water is a good idea. The warm water will help draw blood into your fingertips. Swinging your arm around as if you were throwing a baseball can also draw the blood into your fingertips before pricking your finger.

If you still have trouble getting a good drop of blood, you might try squeezing your finger from your hand outward as if you were "milking" it. Remember to apply a large "hanging" drop of blood to the test area. Smearing the blood on will usually produce a false reading or an "error" message. That means testing all over again and wasting valuable strips. For solutions to other common monitoring mistakes, see Chapter 13: Uncontrolled Diabetes and Sources of Error.

Since test strips can be expensive, it is best to do your test right the first time. And if you want to save money on test strips, order them in bulk through a mail-order pharmacy. This may save you as much as 50% compared to buying them at a retail store. Some meters can also use "generic" test strips (Polymer Technology, Chronimed). These are strips that are made by a company other than the company that makes the meters themselves. Some people have questioned the accuracy of generic test strips, but most studies find that they are equivalent to the more expensive "name brand" strips, and they can save you 20-40% on the cost.

How to become a recording artist.

OK. You have decided to go to the trouble of checking your blood sugar. Now, wouldn't it be a shame to not use all that valuable information you obtain? That's why record keeping is vitally important for everyone with diabetes.

Even your meter's memory cannot replace a good record keeping system. The memory can be useful if you forget to record something on paper, but don't rely on your meter's memory for any more than that.

Generally, it is best to record your readings in four columns: Fasting (pre-breakfast), Pre-Lunch, Pre-Dinner, and Bedtime, plus an area for special notations (see example below):

Date	Breakfast	Lunch	Dinner	Bedtime	Notes
5/21	104	192	67	127	
5/22	109	241	69	115	Had a large breakfast
5/23	113	199	85	105	
5/24	110	211	51	120	Mowed lawn after lunch

This type of system lets you see patterns in your blood sugar levels throughout the day, and can help you to see why your readings may be high or low at certain times. The notes area can be used to describe special situations that may affect your blood sugar levels, such as:

- Stressful events
- Physical activity
- Illness or infection
- Changes from your usual meal plan
- Dining out
- Travel
- Mood changes
- Weather changes
- Injection site changes
- Adjustments to your insulin or medication

In the example above, it is clear that physical activity after lunch can lead to low blood sugar prior to dinner, so a reduction in insulin or increase in food may be in order. And if a large breakfast is planned, an increase in morning insulin or exercise might be necessary. Overall, it also appears that the blood sugar is rising in the morning and falling in the afternoon. If regular and NPH insulin is being taken in the morning, a little more regular and a little less NPH might help stabilize the blood sugar throughout the day.

How often should I test?

Obviously, the more you test, the more you can learn about how different things affect your blood sugar. If you only check your daily fasting (pre-breakfast) blood sugar, you may have a false sense of security. A fasting reading of 110 may be normal, but your blood sugar may be rising to 150 later in the day, and 200 after meals.

Below are <u>monitoring minimums</u> for safe and effective management of your diabetes:

IF YOU DO NOT TAKE PILLS OR INSULIN:

Check your blood sugar at least once a week, ideally first thing in the morning.

IF YOU TAKE PILLS FOR YOUR DIABETES

Cross checking your blood sugar once a day is an excellent way to keep track of your overall blood sugar control. For example:

Sunday	Bedtime
Monday	Before Breakfast
Tuesday	Before Lunch
Wednesday	Before Dinner
Thursday	After Breakfast
Friday	After Lunch
Saturday	After Dinner

CROSS CHECKING

Besides being a rough hockey maneuver, cross checking also means checking your blood sugar at different times each day. This allows you to get a picture of what your blood sugar is like throughout the day without having to check many times each day.

IF YOU TAKE INSULIN OR ARE CHANGING YOUR DOSE OF DIABETES PILLS:

Since your chances of hypoglycemia are greater when you are on insulin or are increasing your medication dosage, more frequent monitoring is necessary. You can use a cross checking pattern, but do two tests a day rather than one:

Sunday	Before Lunch and Bedtime
Monday	Before Breakfast and Dinner
Tuesday	Before Lunch and Bedtime
Wednesday	After Breakfast and Dinner
Thursday	Before Lunch and Bedtime
Friday	Before Breakfast and Lunch
Saturday	After Breakfast and Lunch

ADDITIONAL TIMES TO CHECK

Certain situations will require more frequent monitoring of your blood sugar levels.

Sick Days	**Check every 4-6 hours (you may need supplemental insulin)**
Travel Days	**Check before each meal**
Exercise	**Always check before exercising; check afterward to learn how your body responds. During extended workouts, check every hour.**
Hypoglycemic Unawareness	**Check at least four times a day, and during the night at least once a week.**
Pregnancy	**Check before and after all meals, at bedtime, and during the night.**
High Risk Professions (truck/taxi driving, flying, construction)	**Always check before driving or operating heavy machinery.**
Multiple Insulin Injections, or Insulin Pump Use	**Check before each meal/snack and at bedtime.**

Using blood sugar monitoring to improve your control

The best thing about checking your blood sugar is that you can use the numbers to improve your diabetes control. You can use it immediately to adjust your insulin doses on a sliding scale, or use it to make adjustments the next day to prevent high or low blood sugar from occurring again.

SLIDING SCALE

With a sliding insulin scale, your dosage is adjusted based on your blood sugar level. The higher the reading, the more insulin you take in order to bring the blood sugar back toward normal.

Monitoring is also a valuable learning tool. By analyzing your blood sugar data and the situations under which certain high or low readings occur, you can obtain a wealth of information. For instance, you may come to realize that your blood sugar is lower than usual on hot/humid days, so less insulin is necessary. Or, you may discover that certain exercises lower your blood sugar by different amounts. An hour of tennis may lower your blood sugar by 100 points, but an hour of walking may only lower it by 50. You may need a larger snack (or less insulin) during tennis than during a walk.

Monitoring will teach you that day-to-day activity can also affect your blood sugar levels. One day, your job may have you behind the desk all day, and your blood sugar may tend to run a little on the high side. The next day you find yourself up and about, walking a great deal and carrying things from place to place. As a result, your blood sugar runs low before lunch. Obviously, you will need less insulin (or larger snacks) on active days than on sedentary days.

Through monitoring, you can learn the effect that each unit of insulin has on your blood sugar level. You can estimate this amount by dividing your total daily dose of insulin into 1500. Or, to really find out, take a unit of Humalog or regular when your blood sugar is a little on the high side, don't eat for four hours, and see how much your blood sugar comes down.

You can also find out how much food will be covered by each unit of insulin. This is called an insulin-to-carbohydrate ratio. For example, you may find that if you take three units of regular insulin at breakfast and have 60 grams of carbohydrate, your blood sugar goes up by 60 points by lunch time. Five units causes your blood sugar to go down 40 points. But four units keeps your blood sugar steady from breakfast to lunch. Since 4 units of insulin covers 60 grams of carbohydrate, your insulin-to-carb ratio is 1:15.

Diabetes management is by no means simple. There are countless factors that can affect blood sugar control. However, checking your blood sugar lets you balance the factors that raise and lower your blood sugar. And that is what diabetes management is all about.

Key point:

By checking your blood sugar frequently and using the data to coordinate your meal plan, exercise and pills/insulin, you can greatly improve your diabetes control.

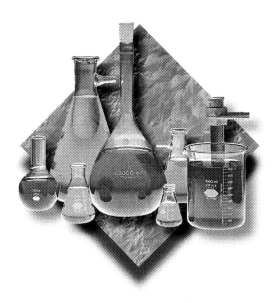

Chapter 11: The Glycosylated Hemoglobin Test

Don't get scared by the name. A glycosylated hemoglobin simply means a red blood cell that has sugar stuck to it, kind of like a doughnut with glazed icing.

Hemoglobin is a special molecule found in the red blood cells. It is responsible for carrying oxygen to different parts of the body. Oxygen sticks to hemoglobin like flies stick to fly paper. And when hemoglobin carries oxygen in the bloodstream, it gives the blood its bright red color.

Sticky Hemoglobin, Sticky Problems

Have you ever spilled something sweet? Makes a sticky mess, doesn't it? Sugar sticks to just about everything - skin, clothes, carpeting, upholstery, your parents' favorite coffee table, you name it. Unfortunately, sugar also sticks to hemoglobin and proteins throughout the body. When the blood sugar level is high, it is like spilling something sweet all over the inside of your body. When sugar starts sticking to proteins, it keeps them from doing their job properly. (If you don't believe it, imagine trying to do your job while coated from head to toe in caramel syrup.)

In particular, sugar will "compete" with oxygen for a place to stick on the hemoglobin molecule. More sugar in the blood means that more hemoglobin molecules will become sugar-coated. Unlike oxygen, which jumps off hemoglobin once it reaches its destination (such as muscle or brain tissue), sugar stays stuck for good. And remember, hemoglobin molecules are embedded in red blood cells, which stay in the blood for about three months. So, by measuring how many hemoglobin molecules have sugar attached, we can estimate how much sugar has been in the blood for the previous three months.

If the blood sugar level has been normal for the past three months, only a small percentage of hemoglobin molecules will have sugar attached. If the blood sugar has been high, a larger percentage will have sugar attached. That is what is meant by "glycosylated hemoglobin" - the percentage of hemoglobin molecules that have sugar attached.

Taking things one step further, it is possible to measure one particular part of the hemoglobin molecule to see if it has sugar attached. This area has been labeled the "A-1-c" area. Thus, a "Hemoglobin A1c" (HbA1c) test is looking at the percentage of hemoglobin molecules that have sugar attached to them at a specific point.

A diabetes control score card

In the DCCT (Diabetes Control and Complications Trial), it was clear that a high HbA1c meant an increased risk for diabetic complications. A lower HbA1c meant less risk of complications. When done regularly, the HbA1c can be a crystal ball into the future.

Remember, an HbA1c test is telling us the percentage of hemoglobin molecules that have sugar attached. This, in turn, correlates with average blood sugar levels over the past three months. When you test your blood sugar with a meter, you are finding out the level at that particular point in time. The HbA1c gives an average of all times for the past three months - before meals, after meals, while you work, while you sleep, during exercise, and so on. Daily blood sugar monitoring is like the number of hits you get in a single baseball game. The glycosylated hemoglobin is like your batting average for the entire season.

If your HbA1c is ...	*Your Average blood sugar for the past 3 months is ...	Risk of Diabetic Complications	Level of Control
4%	60 mg/dl	Very Low	"Normal"
5	90	Very Low	
6	120	Very Low	Tight Diabetic Control
7	150	Low	
8	180	Low	
9	210	Moderate	Poor Diabetic Control
10	240	Moderate	
11	270	High	
12	300	High	
13	330	Very High	
14	360	Very High	

* To calculate your average blood sugar from your HbA1c, multiply the test result by 30 and subtract 60. For example, if your HbA1c is 8.2, your average blood sugar would be 8.2 X 30, or 246, minus 60, which equals 186.

Different tests, different results

It is very important to know that different laboratories do the glyco-sylated hemoglobin test in different ways. While the "normal" range for the HbA1c test is usually 4-6%, some labs may be measuring a part of the hemoglobin molecule other than the A1c portion. As a result, the normal range could by 4-8%, 5-7%, 6-8%, or 5-9%. A score of 9.1 on a test with a normal range of 6-8 could mean pretty good control, but if the normal range is 4-6, a 9.1 could mean rather poor control.

Always ask your doctor for the normal range on the test you are taking along with your test result. Your doctor can help you interpret your score based on the normal range and your scores on previous tests.

About the test itself...

Since the glycosylated hemoglobin gives a three-month average of blood sugar control, people who take insulin should have the test performed every three months. If you just take pills or control your diabetes through diet and exercise, it should be taken every 6 to 12 months. During pregnancy, the test should be performed every month.

The "preferred form" of the test is the HbA1c since this is the test that was used in the DCCT study. However, any glycosylated hemoglobin test will provide valuable data.

It is not necessary to fast for a glycosylated hemoglobin test, so it may be performed at any time of day. If you take large doses of Vitamin C or Vitamin E, the test result may be falsely low. This is because Vitamins C and E may prevent sugar from sticking to the hemoglobin molecules.

Interpreting the result

It is important to remember that the glycosylated hemoglobin test does not take the place of routine testing of your blood sugar. Daily blood sugar tests are still necessary for you to make decisions about your meal plan, exercise, and insulin/medication doses. By using the data from your own monitoring, you can improve your score on your next glycosylated hemoglobin test.

If your glycosylated hemoglobin is in a "tight" or "normal" range, you may or may not have good control of your diabetes. Remember, the test is an average of all your blood sugar levels for the past three months. Ask yourself, "Did I have a lot of low blood sugars?" If you did, your control may not be as good as you might think. After all, readings of 50 and 250 average out to 150, just the same as readings of 125 and 175 average out to 150. Obviously, fewer "highs and lows" means more stable blood sugars, less risk of severe hypoglycemia, and better overall control. It is better to run blood sugars of 125 and 175 than to have constant highs of 250 and lows of 50.

If your glycosylated hemoglobin is high, you might consider making a change to your current diabetes management plan. You may need to exercise more or cut down on your food. You may need to increase your dosage of insulin or medication, or start taking them for the first time. More frequent blood sugar monitoring will help you to find out where the trouble is. Perhaps your blood sugar is going very high after meals or snacks, during the night, or early in the morning.

Remember, your average readings taken from blood sugar monitoring are usually going to be less than the average taken from your glycosylated hemoglobin test. Most blood sugar readings are taken before meals, when the blood sugar is at its lowest point. The glycosylated hemoglobin also includes blood sugar levels after meals, when readings tend to be higher.

The glycosylated hemoglobin is a valuable tool for assessing your overall blood sugar control. Use it in conjunction with your daily monitoring to find out how well your overall control is and how close you are to reaching your diabetes management goals.

Key Point:

The glycosylated hemoglobin test, also called a HbA1c, tells the average blood sugar level for the previous three months.

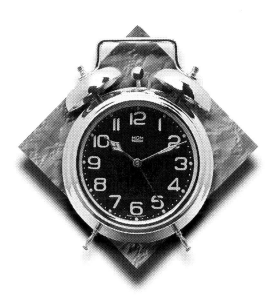

Chapter 12:
Intensifying Control & Making Adjustments

Intensive management. Sounds like one of those weekend courses designed to help you get ahead in business. In this case, intensive management means tight blood sugar control - readings as close to normal as possible, as much of the time as possible.

So why not just keep the levels low all the time? There is a trade-off: Lower blood sugars means less risk of complications, but it also means a greater risk of serious hypoglycemia.

Intensive control does not mean perfect blood sugar levels. We like to define it as: **A diabetes management plan that significantly lowers your risk of long-term complications and improves your quality of** life, but without putting you at risk for severe hypoglycemia. In other words, it is better to have your blood sugar levels be 100 before meals and 180 after rather than 50 before and 150 after, or 150 before and 250 after.

The Balancing Act

To achieve intensive control of your diabetes, you will need to balance the factors that raise blood sugar with those that lower blood sugar. Readings that are too high or too low mean that there is an imbalance - the scales are not even. It will be up to you to figure out where the imbalance exists and how to make things balance out. That is what diabetes management is all about.

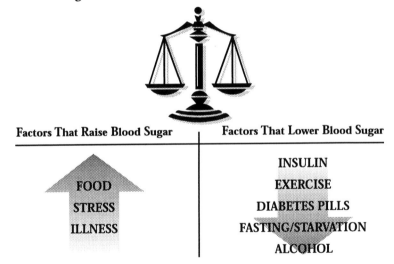

Factors That Raise Blood Sugar	Factors That Lower Blood Sugar
FOOD	INSULIN
STRESS	EXERCISE
ILLNESS	DIABETES PILLS
	FASTING/STARVATION
	ALCOHOL

Goal Setting

Making changes in our lifestyle habits and general way of doing things is never easy. It is best to take "small steps" toward your goal rather than trying to do everything at once.

Level of Control	Fasting/Pre-Meal	2 Hrs. After Meal	Bedtime	HbA1c
Very Intense	70 - 120	<150	80 - 140	6 - 7
Intense	70 - 150	<180	100 - 150	7 - 8
Loose	120 - 200	<240	120 - 240	8 - 10
Poor	>200	>300	>200	>10

For instance, if your control now is poor, it probably would not be wise to jump to very intense control all of a sudden. You would probably be overwhelmed with all the changes you need to make, and might have some serious low blood sugars along the way. It is best to move up a stage at a time - from poor to loose, from loose to intense, intense to very intense.

When setting goals, begin with a few immediate habit changes (described in the sections that follow) and set short-term goals with 3-6 months to achieve them. For example, immediate actions are to take your regular insulin at least 30 minutes prior to meals or exercise each morning after breakfast. Your short term goal might be to lower your HbA1c from 9 to 8, or have 75% of your blood sugar readings between 80 and 180. Whatever immediate actions and short term goals you choose, WRITE THEM DOWN and post them someplace where you will see them often - such as a bathroom mirror or refrigerator.

Conventional vs. Intensive Therapy

Webster's dictionary defines "conventional" as "established, but lacking originality or individuality." Let's face it. If it lacks originality and individuality, it's not going to work very well.

When it comes to treating diabetes, conventional therapy means one or two shots of insulin a day, usually NPH or Lente, possibly mixed with regular insulin. Blood sugars are checked once or twice daily, mainly to let the doctor know how the insulin program is working. Conventional therapy is convenient but hardly flexible, and definitely not ideal for achieving the best possible blood sugar control. After all, NPH in the morning means that most of your day has to be according to schedule. Deviate from that schedule, and blood sugars can go very high or very low. You pretty much eat the same amount of food, get the same amount of activity, and take the same insulin doses day-in and day-out. The person with diabetes has very little decision-making power.

Intensive therapy puts the person with diabetes in the driver's seat. Insulin doses, food intake and activity levels can vary depending on the individual's needs and lifestyle. The key element of intensive therapy is education. Each person must learn how to make adjustments in order to keep the blood sugar from going too high or too low. Using our earlier analogy, the two sides of the scale must be kept in balance: the factors raising the blood sugar should equal the factors that lower it.

Through intensive therapy, you can expect to achieve tighter blood sugar control and have a lower HbA1c. You will also have more flexibility due to the ability to make adjustments for day-to-day meals and activities. And even though your blood sugar will be lower overall, your risk of hypoglycemia may actually be reduced on intensive therapy. Remember, on conventional therapy, any delay in a meal, reduced meal size or unexpected activity will usually lead to low blood sugar. With intensive therapy, you can make adjustments to prevent hypoglycemia before it happens.

Checklist for intensive therapy

For intensive therapy to work well and give you all the benefits described above, certain things are essential:

• EDUCATION - You must be well informed and motivated. Keeping up to date on the latest technology and methods of diabetes management will let you stay on top of your control. Read all you can (JDF's Countdown, ADA's Diabetes Forecast, Rapaport's Diabetes Self-Management, Kings Publishing's Diabetes Interview - see Appendix B), attend diabetes management classes and seminars, and ask your doctor and diabetes educators to teach you about how to better control your diabetes.

• CARB COUNTING - Since carbohydrates in the diet are the major factor that increases blood sugar, knowing the amount of carbohydrate in your food can allow you to make sensible insulin dosage adjustments and regulate your blood sugar effectively. Many people choose to determine an "insulin-to-carbs" ratio that suits them best. For example, you may need 1 unit of insulin for every 15 grams of carbohydrate. A meal containing 60 grams of carbohydrate will require 4 units of insulin in order to keep the blood sugar within range several hours later. Even if you don't adjust your insulin doses, figuring the appropriate amount of carbohydrate for each meal can produce consistent blood sugar levels. For more information on carbohydrate counting, see Chapter 4.

• AVOIDANCE OF LOW BLOOD SUGAR - Low blood sugar gives you two headaches for the price of one. First, the low blood sugar can be dangerous if not treated quickly and appropriately. Second, low blood sugar is often followed by a high blood sugar - the result of the liver's slow but significant efforts to raise the blood sugar level, or possibly overtreatment of hypoglycemia with too much food. In either case, the result can be a rollercoaster of low readings, followed by high, followed by low, etc. Prevention of low blood sugar involves appropriate meal timing and carbohydrate content of meals; insulin dosage or snack adjustments for exercise and physical activity; and treating high readings conservatively - i.e. not overtreating high readings with too much insulin. For more details, see the following chapter.

• FREQUENT MONITORING - As Chapter 10 covered in detail, blood sugar monitoring is an important part of intensive therapy. By knowing your blood sugar at key junctures during the day and night, you can make intelligent decisions that will keep (or get) your blood sugar levels in a healthy range. Blood sugar should be checked prior to each meal and at bedtime every day. It should be checked two hours after meals on a rotating basis (breakfast one day, lunch the next, dinner the next, breakfast the next, etc.). It should be checked at least once a month at 3 a.m. to confirm that your blood sugar is not dropping too low during the night. Checking before exercise (and after, when first starting an exercise program) will let you see how you respond to exercise, and what type of food or insulin adjustments need to be made.

• GOOD RECORD KEEPING - Just keeping track of your blood sugar readings is not enough. It is most important to know what caused high and low readings, not just when they took place. Along with your blood sugars, keep track of your insulin doses, carbohydrate intake, physical activity, and any unusual factors (such as stress or illness) that might impact your blood sugar levels.

• MULTIPLE INSULIN INJECTIONS - By taking multiple doses of fast-acting insulin before meals, along with an intermediate or long-acting insulin through the night, you are "copying" what your pancreas tries to do. That is, increasing the insulin level when you need it (after meals), and keeping the level low when you don't need it (between meals and while you sleep). Consider one of the following insulin programs:

R = Regular Insulin N = NPH or Lente Insulin H = Humalog U = Ultralente Insulin	BENEFITS	DRAWBACKS
• N and R in the morning • R at dinner • N at bedtime	• Breakfast and Dinner can vary. • Low risk of hypoglycemia during the night. • Nighttime N helps cover early morning dawn effect.	• Lunch and afternoon activities must be on schedule. • Mid-morning snack may be necessary.
• N and H in the morning • H at dinner • N at bedtime	• Breakfast and Dinner can vary. • Low risk of hypoglycemia during the night. • Nighttime N helps cover early morning dawn effect. • Better control after breakfast and dinner.	• Lunch and afternoon activities must be on schedule. • Dinner and bedtime shots must be within 4 hours of each other.
• R before breakfast, lunch, dinner • N at bedtime	• All meals can vary.	• Snacking may be necessary 3 hours after R. • 4 injections a day.
• H before breakfast, lunch, dinner • N at bedtime	• All meals can vary. • Better control after meals.	• Blood sugary may rise before meals due to short action of H. • 4 injections a day.
• R before breakfast, lunch, dinner • U at dinner, or breakfast & dinner	• All meals can vary. • 3 injections a day.	• Snacking between meals may be necessary.
• H before breakfast, lunch, dinner • U at dinner, or breakfast & dinner	• All meals can vary. • 3 injections a day • Better control after meals.	
• Insulin Pump Therapy (continuous basal insulin infusion, plus bolus of fast-acting insulin before meals and snacks)	• No shots. • Offers most flexibility. • All meals can vary. • Can vary times of meals, activities.	• Must wear pump continuously. • Must change infusion set every 2-3 days.

Making Insulin Adjustments

When making adjustments to insulin doses, it is important to remember two things:

First, if you have Type-I diabetes, never let your body run out of insulin completely. Doing so can cause your blood sugar to rise very high and lead to a life-threatening condition called ketoacidosis (see chapter 14). In other words, if you only take short-acting insulins during the day and have no long-acting insulin in the "background", skipping or delaying a dose could cause you to run out of insulin completely and lead to some serious problems.

Second, it is important to remember which insulin works when. Humalog insulin peaks 1-2 hours after it is taken, so it will only cover the meal you are about to eat. Regular insulin peaks in 2-4 hours, so it will cover an upcoming meal and possibly a snack later on. NPH and Lente peak in 4-8 hours, so a breakfast shot will cover lunch; a dinner shot will cover bedtime; and a bedtime shot will cover the early morning hours. Ultralente does not have a distinct peak action time, so it serves as a "background insulin".

Let's look at the following example for Lisa, who takes Regular and NPH in the morning, regular at dinner, and NPH at bedtime:

Date	Breakfast (4R,20N)	Lunch	Dinner (6R)	Bedtime (12N)	Notes
5/21	104	192	67	*127	*Exercised after dinner
5/22	129	241	69	*115	Large breakfast *Exercised
5/23	113	199	85	195	No exercise
5/24	140	211	51	120	Mowed lawn after lunch

In this example, the morning regular insulin (4R) covers breakfast, so the lunchtime reading reflects how well this dose of insulin worked. The morning NPH (20N) covers lunch, so the dinnertime reading reflects how well the NPH worked. The dinnertime regular (6R) covers dinner, so the bedtime reading reflects how well the regular worked. Finally, the bedtime NPH (12N) covers the bedtime snack and the liver's release of sugar through the night, so the morning reading reflects how well the NPH worked.

What do you notice from looking at Lisa's readings?

First, you might notice that Lisa's blood sugar tends to go up from breakfast to lunch. This indicates that the morning dose of regular was not enough to cover the food that was eaten. To make her blood sugar balance better, she could either eat less or take more insulin. Since Lisa enjoys her standard bagel & eggs breakfast, our only other choice is to increase her dose of morning regular insulin. By increasing it to six units, her lunchtime readings should come down toward normal.

You might also notice that her blood sugar comes down a great deal between lunch and dinner. If her lunchtime readings are going to be lower (with her larger dose of regular in the morning), it would be dangerous to have such a large blood sugar drop in the afternoon. The logical decision would be to either eat more food, exercise less, or take less NPH in the morning. Since Lisa prefers to exercise in the evening and does not want to gain weight, her preference is to lower her morning NPH dose. By lowering her dose to 16 units, she should be able to avoid low blood sugar before dinner.

Next, you might have noticed that Lisa's bedtime blood sugar is excellent if she exercises in the evening, but goes pretty high when she gets no physical activity. To correct this, Lisa decided to increase her dinner time dose of regular to 8 units if she doesn't plan to exercise. By doing this, her bedtime readings should be consistently in the normal range.

What about Lisa's nighttime readings? It appears that her morning readings are pretty close to what her reading was the night before. This indicates that her bedtime NPH is probably set properly.

Finally, from looking at the "notes" section, we notice that Lisa's blood sugar went very high after a "large" breakfast (there was a 2-for-1 sale at the bagel shop). From this, we learn that Lisa must be careful to limit her carbohydrate intake in the morning, or she can wind up severely hyperglycemic. Or, if she chooses to eat more than usual, she will need to take extra regular insulin in the morning.

The low dinnertime reading on 5/24 was likely due to Lisa's lawn mowing. She now knows to treat yardwork the same as exercise. The next time she mows the lawn in the afternoon, she plans to either eat an extra piece of fruit at lunch or lower her morning NPH by 2 units.

The insulin adjustments described above are called pattern adjustments. They are made in response to consistent changes seen in blood sugar levels. Pattern adjustments cannot correct a high or low reading

---

PATTERN ADJUSTMENT
The art of adjusting insulin doses based on consistently high or low readings in order to prevent such readings in the future.

---

immediately, but they can prevent the problem from happening again. In general, if you experience readings that are out of range for two or three consecutive days, consider your options: Are you eating too much or too little carbohydrate? Is your physical activity excessive or too little? Or does your insulin need to be adjusted? If you conclude that your insulin needs adjustment, make the change in small increments of 20% or less, and see how this works. If more adjustment is needed, then adjust by another 20%. It is always best to change only one insulin at a time. A change in one insulin can affect the body's need for insulin at other times of day.

SLIDING SCALE
The art of making a one-time insulin dosage adjustment to immediately correct a high or low reading.

Another way of adjusting insulin doses is by what is called a "sliding scale" method. No, it has nothing to do with throwing your bathroom scale across the floor to see how many syringes you can knock down. A sliding scale means that your insulin dose is based on what your blood sugar is at the time of your injection. In Lisa's case, she could vary her breakfast and dinner doses of regular according to the following scale:

If pre-meal blood sugar is...	Take this much insulin...
<80	5 units
80 -150	6 units
150 - 200	7 units
200 - 250	8 units
250 - 300	9 units
>300	10 units

Her evening dose of NPH could be based on a different sliding scale:

If bedtime blood sugar is...	Take this much insulin...
<80	10 units
80 - 200	12 units
>200	14 units

A sliding scale is a fast way to correct a reading that is too high or too low, but it will not prevent the problem from happening again. That is why pattern adjustment should be used along with the sliding scale to lower the HbA1c and achieve the best overall control.

Tips for controlling blood sugar after meals

The HbA1c is an equal-opportunity lab test. It doesn't care when the blood sugar is high. If it is high at any time, it will be factored into your test result, and ultimately into your risk for complications.

POSTPRANDIAL BLOOD SUGAR

This is another way of saying "blood sugar within four hours after eating a meal."

Because of this, we cannot ignore the importance of keeping blood sugars controlled after meals. Your fasting and pre-meal blood sugars will almost always be lower than your postprandial readings by up to 100 or even 200 points. It is not uncommon to have a fasting reading of 110 that goes up to 280 after breakfast. Of course, the first step in controlling postprandial readings is to keep the pre-meal levels in good control. A pre-meal value of 210 will almost always lead to a higher postprandial value than a pre-meal value of 110.

Below are a few techniques that can help you manage your postprandial blood sugar levels:

- FIBER: Adding fiber to your diet will slow the absorption of sugar from the digestive tract.

- GLUCOTROL: Glucotrol is one of the OHAs (sulfonylureas) that lowers blood sugar after meals.

- GLUCOPHAGE: By improving cellular sensitivity to insulin, Glucophage helps blood sugar levels come down faster after meals.

- HUMALOG: This fast-acting insulin works better than regular insulin for controlling postprandial blood sugar levels.

- EXERCISE: Exercising 30-60 minutes after a meal will help minimize the postprandial rise in blood sugar.

- PRECOSE: By slowing the digestion of carbohydrates, Precose lowers postprandial blood sugars by an average of 50 points.

Intensive Management in Type-II Diabetes

Intensive management is not just for those lucky enough to have Type-I diabetes. If you have Type-II, there is plenty you can do to improve your blood sugar control. Regardless of the severity of your diabetes, you can apply the "balancing" principles given above. Look for ways to make the factors that raise your blood sugar (food, stress, illness) equal the factors that lower your blood sugar (activity, insulin, diabetes pills).

If you already take insulin two or more times a day, you can probably follow the general recommendations given earlier in this chapter for intensive therapy. However, if you are on one shot a day, diabetes pills, or no medication at all, and your control is less than ideal, don't sit idly by assuming that everything is okay. If your HbA1c is above 7.1, or if your fasting or pre-meal blood sugars are over 120, your control is not what it could or should be. You probably have less energy than you should and may be going to the bathroom during the night, not to mention that you are putting yourself at high risk for the long-term complications of diabetes. THE TIME IS NOW TO DO SOMETHING ABOUT IT! You simply cannot wait, because your health depends on it.

1. <u>If you are not taking any pills or insulin for your diabetes</u>, first ask yourself whether you have made a serious attempt to exercise, follow a healthy meal plan and lose weight. If you have, it is time to consider a diabetes medication, such as Precose or Glucophage, with or without a sulfonylurea (OHA).

2. <u>If you are taking sulfonylureas (OHA) now</u>, it may be time to add Glucophage. Research has shown that the combination of OHA and Glucophage can be much more powerful than each medication taken individually. Precose may also help improve your control, especially after meals.

3. <u>If you are taking Glucophage and/or a maximum dose of OHA</u>, it may be time to start taking insulin. If your morning readings are above normal, the combination of daytime OHA and nighttime NPH insulin can be very effective. If the thought of using a needle is keeping you from taking the insulin your body needs, consider using one of the needle-free insulin injectors (Health-Mor's AdvantaJet, MediJect's MediJector - see Appendix B).

4. <u>If you are already taking nighttime insulin but your daytime readings are high</u>, it is probably time to start taking insulin in the morning - either a single dose of NPH or NPH and regular, or possibly a pre-mixed insulin such as 70/30.

Remember, the only constant in this world is change. <u>Type-II diabetes is a progressive illness that will require more potent forms of therapy as time goes on.</u> IT IS NOT YOUR FAULT if your blood sugar control worsens. You were simply blessed with a bum pancreas. But if you are the type that refuses to accept change and rejects any attempts to adapt to your body's needs, you are going to be in for some serious problems.

Think back to when you were younger, getting your first job, going away to school, getting married, or having your first baby. Remember all the changes you faced and adjusting you had to do just to make it through? Diabetes is no different.

Learn to roll with the punches. It's your ticket to success... and survival.

Key Point:

Intensive control of blood sugar levels is achievable through proper training and the ability to make sound decisions about your day-to-day control.

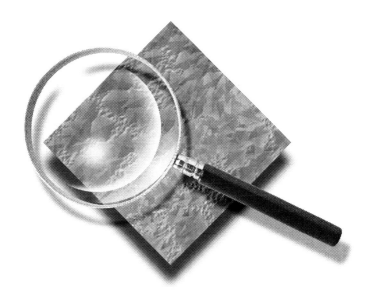

Chapter 13: Sources of Uncontrolled Diabetes: Explaining the Unexplainable

Diabetes management is not a perfect science. Sometimes it may even feel like you're in the Twilight Zone. You think you're doing the same things day after day, but your blood sugar levels go up and down, seemingly without reason.

The purpose of this chapter is to find the reasons — and if we look hard enough, we can almost always find them. There are many things that can change your blood sugar levels. Unfortunately, most people don't have the time, patience or expertise to uncover the real causes of blood sugar variations, so we simply call it "brittle diabetes". If you want to know the truth, "brittle diabetes" simply means that the blood sugar goes up and down for reasons that you and your doctor have yet to figure out.

So, what is it that keeps us from achieving stable, consistent blood sugar levels? There can be literally thousands of factors that play a role, depending on your specific lifestyle and self-care practices. Below are some of the common causes of poor blood sugar control, and steps you can take to achieve better control.

Incorrect rotation of injection sites

For consistent insulin absorption, inject the same body parts from day to day.

Insulin injected in the same spot several days in a row tends to damage the tissue under the skin. Insulin injected in that site is going to be absorbed more slowly than usual, resulting in less insulin reaching the bloodstream. The result, as you can guess, is higher-than-usual blood sugar levels. By moving your injection sites at least one inch each time you give an injection, you can prevent this problem from occurring.

Another variable is the rate of insulin absorption that we get from injecting different parts of the body. If you take your morning shot in the abdomen (stomach) one day, the arm the next day, and the leg the next day, the rate at which the insulin is absorbed will be very different each day. The result: your blood sugar two hours after eating could be very high one day, normal the next day, and low the next. To eliminate this problem, use the same body part for each time of day. For example, always use your abdomen in the morning, leg in the evening, and buttocks at bedtime. Consistency is the key to success!

Technical problems with insulin injections

Drawing up and injecting insulin is a complex procedure, but one which we can all master. Common mistakes made when taking insulin include:

1) Reading the number markings incorrectly (a MagniGuide magnifier or insulin pen with audible clicks can help overcome this).

2) Large air bubbles in the syringe (drawing some insulin into the syringe and pushing it back into the bottle before drawing out your actual dose can prevent air bubbles)

3) Mixing insulins in the wrong order (the clear insulin should always be drawn into the syringe first to prevent contamination)

4) Forgetting to pinch the skin (pinching the skin makes sure the insulin goes into the fat tissue below the skin, and not into the muscle where it may be absorbed too fast)

5) Forgetting to roll the bottle before injecting (if the contents of the bottle are not mixed evenly, you may not get the insulin at full strength)

6) Getting the insulins mixed up; i.e. taking the right dosage, but using the wrong bottle (marking your fast acting insulin with a string or long piece of tape can help prevent this error)

If you continue to have problems giving yourself insulin injections, there are a number of devices that can help: The Inject-Ease insulin injector; the InsulCap (for directing the needle into the vial of insulin correctly), the MagniGuide (for enlarging the numbers on the syringe), the insulin pen (a pre-filled insulin syringe that allows you to simply "dial up" a dose), or you may consider switching to a needle-free insulin injector such as the MediJector or AdvantaJet.

Spoiled insulin

In some cases, rising blood sugar levels can be attributed to insulin that has gone bad or has simply lost its potency. Here is what you can do to prevent this from happening to you:

1) It is OK to keep your insulin at room temperature, but start a new vial each month.

2) Store your unused vials of insulin in the refrigerator.

3) Check the expiration date printed on the box and the vial. Do not use insulin after the expiration date.

4) Once you have started using a vial of insulin, discard it after one month. Using a fresh vial each month will help maintain your insulin at full strength.

5) It is OK to keep your vial of insulin at room temperature (below 86 degrees Fahrenheit) once it has been opened. Do not expose your insulin to extreme heat, freezing cold, or direct sunlight. Leaving your insulin in the car is asking for trouble.

6) Do not use insulin that appears to have something wrong with it. If it has crystals on the surface, does not mix uniformly, has residue at the bottom even after mixing or has an unusual color, it has probably gone bad and should be thrown away.

Infection

You may require a larger insulin dose while fighting infection.

Infection anywhere in the body — from a common sinus infection to a major foot ulcer — can cause blood sugar levels to be higher than usual. The body responds to infection by signaling the liver to release extra glucose into the bloodstream. Unfortunately, high blood sugar can actually impair the body's ability to fight infection. So, to keep your diabetes under control and speed your recovery from infection, work with your doctor on adjusting your dosage of insulin or medication, and monitor more frequently.

Gastroparesis

Gastroparesis is a form of diabetic neuropathy (nerve disease) in which food is digested slower than it should be. People with gastroparesis usually feel full, and they may experience nausea, vomiting, or stomach pain after eating. When gastroparesis acts up, blood sugar does not rise very much after a meal — but it may rise several hours later as food begins to be digested. Gasatroparesis requires that you work closely with your physician to manage your blood sugar levels.

For those trying to achieve tight blood sugar control, gastroparesis can be a source of great frustration. All you learned about the relationship between food and insulin may be backwards: Blood sugar may actually go down after eating, and then go up before the next meal.

Gastroparesis can be treated with drugs that help promote digestion, such as Reglan or Propulsid. It is best to eat frequent, small meals rather than a few large meals. Because fiber tends to slow down digestion even more, people with gastroparesis may benefit from a low fiber diet (cutting down on fruits, vegetables and whole grains). For those who take regular insulin prior to meals, it can be beneficial to take the insulin after rather than before the meal. That way, the insulin will peak at about the same time that the food is being absorbed into the bloodstream.

Diabetus Overwhelmus

When you have a complex, never-ending disease such as diabetes, it is easy to become overwhelmed and simply stop doing the things you need to do to keep it under control. Perhaps other things in your life are taking precedence. Or maybe your doctor is trying to get you to do too much all at once.

In any case, start out by accepting that we can't be perfect. **IT IS OK** to "fall off the wagon" from time to time. It's what makes us human. Trust in yourself that when you're ready, you'll get right back on, and maybe even try to do things a little better than before. And if a lot of diabetes management is new to you, take it in small, manageable chunks. Once you've mastered a particular area, you're ready to add to your knowledge and skills. Trying to make many changes all at once can lead to mistakes, frustration, and errors in judgment.

Forgetting to adjust for physical activity

It should be ingrained in your brain by now that exercise lowers blood sugar levels. It does this by making insulin more efficient; each molecule of insulin gets more sugar out of the bloodstream and into cells when you exercise.

But did you know that <u>any</u> extra physical activity can make your insulin work better? That includes everyday things like walking the dog, planting petunias, sweeping the floor, or even having sex. Anything that has you using your muscles in a repetitive manner will tend to bring your blood sugar down.

Rich, for example, has good blood sugar control throughout the week, except for Sunday mornings. "I can't figure it out," he said. "I have my usual breakfast, take my usual amount of insulin, and just relax by doing some yardwork."

Bingo! By not reducing his insulin when he did yardwork, Rich was consistently getting low blood sugar. One small adjustment was all it took to correct the problem.

Ohmygod!!! Stress!!!

Stress can cause an immediate and severe rise in blood sugar levels.

According to psychological research, the thing that causes people the greatest amount of stress is speaking in front of an audience.

Recently, a colleague put this theory to the test. Several hours prior to going in front of an audience to sing and play guitar in public for the first time, his blood sugar was a modest 130. As the evening approached, he was noticeably nervous. He didn't eat, didn't move around much, and spent a lot of time in the bathroom. Just before going on stage, he did another blood sugar check. Three hundred and ten.

Just goes to show what a little stress can do. Stress can take many forms, from physical stresses such as spraining an ankle, to psychological stresses such as test anxiety or fighting traffic. Whatever the cause, stress can produce an immediate and severe rise in blood sugar levels. The problem is that stress is usually unpredictable. But when it is predictable, such as when we know that the in-laws are coming to visit or that a big game is coming up, we can adjust our food intake, insulin/medication, or physical activity ahead of time to compensate for it.

Our friend with the guitar now gives himself almost twice as much NPH insulin the morning of a presentation as he takes on a normal day. He still can't carry a tune to save his life, but his blood sugar has certainly improved.

Overtreatment of low blood sugar

It is easy to become a "remorseless eating machine" when your blood sugar is low. After all, the cure for the shakes is sugar. And when you've got the shakes, it can be tempting to keep eating until those shakes go away.

But here's the catch. Do that, and you're almost guaranteed to have a blood sugar in the 200s, 300s or 400s a couple of hours later. As if the low blood sugar wasn't frustrating enough, now you have a high blood sugar (with the extra thirst, urinating, tiredness and appetite) to deal with.

Instead of creating two problems for the price of one, it makes much more sense to treat the low blood sugar right in the first place. Limit your intake to 15-30 grams of carbohydrate (depending on the severity of your hypoglycemia), and then Be Patient. Give your blood sugar 15 to 30 minutes to come up. If you don't think you can keep your face out of the refrigerator, keep yourself occupied by reading a magazine, playing solitaire, or watching TV.

Chasing high blood sugar

Here's another way to create two problems for the price of one. When your blood sugar is high, give yourself lots of insulin to bring it down. Maybe even take the insulin and then do some exercise to help bring it down faster. Either way, you're probably headed straight for low-blood-sugarsville.

Often, people forget that it takes 4-6 hours for regular insulin to exert its full effects, and 10-12 hours for NPH and Lente insulins to do the same. If you check your blood sugar 2 hours after eating and find that it is too high, at least give the insulin you took prior to the meal a chance to work. If it is still high four hours after eating, you can bring it down by taking supplemental insulin according to the "1500 rule" (see below). More importantly, <u>try to prevent the problem from happening again by adjusting your pre-meal dose the next day</u>.

"1500 Rule"

If the total amount of insulin you take in a day is this...	Each extra unit of insulin will lower you by this much...
10 units	150 points
15 units	100 points
20 units	75 points
25 units	60 points
30 units	50 points
35 units	43 points
40 units	38 points
45 units	33 points
50 units	30 points
60 units	25 points
75 units	20 points
100 units	15 points
150 units	10 points

Inconsistent carb intake

Anyone who has had diabetes for many years knows how the dietary rules have changed. It used to be that a person with diabetes could eat an unlimited amount of bread and potatoes, but cake and candy were strictly forbidden. Today, we understand that most carbohydrates — whether they come in the form of starch or simple sugar — tend to raise the blood sugar by similar amounts. In other words, a carb is a carb is a carb.

Take the case of Betty. Some days, Betty has what would be considered a "healthy" breakfast: A big bowl of cereal, a bagel, a cup of orange juice, and a cup of milk. However, on some days, she is in a hurry and barely has time to grab a doughnut and a cup of coffee. The thing is, Betty's blood sugar is much higher after the "healthy" breakfast than after the quickie doughnut. Why? Because the healthy breakfast contains over 100 grams of carbohydrate, while the doughnut and coffee contains only about 30 grams. Sure, the doughnut and coffee provide very little nutrition and may contain a great deal of fat, but the effect on blood sugar depends primarily on the carbohydrate content of the meal.

Now, when Betty has time to sit down for breakfast, she has the same cereal, but with a half cup of milk and juice, and no bagel. When she's in a hurry, she grabs a breakfast bar and a banana. Because both breakfasts contain about 50 grams of carbohydrate, her mid-morning and pre-lunch blood sugar levels are more stable and consistent than they were before.

Count the amount of carbohydrate in your meals and snacks, and try to be consistent from day to day. Read the food labels, and measure your portion sizes to see how much you're actually having. Talk to a dietitian if you would like to learn to count carbohydrates accurately. And if you find yourself having more or less than usual, you may need to adjust your insulin or activity level to keep your blood sugar under control.

Fat and Protein

Although carbohydrate plays the major role in raising blood sugar levels, large amounts of fat and protein may also cause blood sugar to rise. A small percentage of the fat and protein we eat gets converted into sugar during digestion. This conversion usually takes several hours to occur. Therefore, a meal high in fat or protein, such as a large steak or buttery popcorn, can cause high blood sugar several hours after it is eaten.

To compensate for high fat or protein intake, try exercising a few hours after your meal, or increase your pre-meal NPH or Lente insulin by 10%. If these adjustments fail to bring your blood sugar down, try a longer workout or a 20% insulin increase next time, or take a small dose of regular insulin a few hours after eating.

Meal Composition

It is a fact that fat, protein and fiber can slow down the digestion of carbohydrates. By including these nutrients in your meals, you can effectively delay the rise in blood sugar that normally occurs after eating.

The opposite is also true. Meals that contain mostly carbohydrates will lead to the quickest and largest rise in blood sugar. Pizza, for example, will probably drive your blood sugar up very fast if eaten by itself. Combine it with a large salad, however, and the rise in blood sugar will probably be smaller and slower.

Somogyi effect

No, it's not something out of a 1950s Japanese monster movie. The Somogyi effect, also called a "rebound effect," means high blood sugar that occurs in response to low blood sugar.

When we become hypoglycemic, we also produce two hormones intended to drive the sugar back up: adrenaline and glucagon. This is nature's way of protecting us from getting very low blood sugar. The most common time for this to occur is during the night while we sleep. That's why a moderately low blood sugar during the night can actually result in high blood sugar the following morning!

Take the case of Jessie. For several days in a row, Jessie woke up at 7 a.m. with blood sugar in the 200s. She always checked her blood at bedtime, and it was never over 150. What could be causing the problem? To figure it out, Jessie set her alarm for 3 a.m. the next night, and checked her blood sugar. What she found amazed her. It was only 55! Apparently, Jessie was either taking too much insulin at night, or not having enough to eat at bedtime. She chose to cut back on her nighttime NPH insulin by 10%, and the problem went away.

Imagine! Taking less insulin actually brought her morning blood sugar down. Without checking her 3 a.m. blood sugar, she might have assumed that she wasn't taking enough insulin at night, and would have started taking even more. Of course, that would have made the problem worse.

The Somogyi effect can keep the blood sugar high for up to 10 hours, so it is very important to test and see if it is happening to you. In addition to doing a nighttime blood sugar test, symptoms that may indicate low blood sugar during the night include:

- nighttime sweating
- cool body temperature
- restlessness
- headache/hangover-like symptoms
- rapid heart rate
- nightmares
- not feeling well-rested in the morning

Timing of meals and insulin

Our mission is to match the insulin peak to our food absorption.

With the development of newer and faster-acting insulins, this becomes easier to accomplish. Ideally we want to have the insulin starting to peak at about the same time our food is being digested and absorbed into the bloodstream. That way, the forces raising and lowering the blood sugar will balance out, and the blood sugar should not go too high or too low after eating.

In general, if your blood sugar is within a good range (as determined by you and your doctor) prior to a meal, you should try to take your regular insulin 30 minutes before eating, and Humalog (lyspro) insulin 10 minutes before eating. If your blood sugar is low prior to the meal, take your insulin and eat right away, starting with 15-30 grams of carbohydrate to bring your blood sugar up.

When the pre-meal blood sugar is high, we need to wait longer after taking the shot. Insulin does not work as well or as quickly when the blood sugar is high. High blood sugar also increases the appetite. It may be tempting to eat soon after taking your insulin, but try to resist the temptation. If your blood sugar is too high, give your regular insulin an hour before eating, and your Humalog insulin 30 minutes before eating.

Attention-getting maneuvers

If someone you know has blood sugar levels that bounce around like a rubber ball, they may be seeking attention for issues that are completely unrelated to their diabetes. A child may be frustrated with his parents. He may feel suffocated, neglected or abused. Or he may be having problems adjusting to life with diabetes. In any case, he may see a trip to the hospital or doctor's office as an opportunity to receive gifts, attention, or a safe refuge.

Adults, particularly older adults, may experience similar feelings from time to time. Marital problems, loneliness, money issues, or difficulties coping with the aging process can prompt almost anyone to seek attention and a kind listening ear.

Trying to control blood sugar before fixing these underlying problems is like trying to pull a weed out by the leaves. If the root is not removed, the weed will just keep growing back. Get to the root cause of the problem first.

Insomnia

Being awake at night, in and of itself, does not have an adverse effect on blood sugar levels. It's what we do while we're awake that can create problems.

Most of us read or watch TV when we can't fall asleep. We also munch... on pretzels, potato chips, popcorn, or whatever we can get our hands on. All that extra munching not only causes weight gain, it causes high blood sugar.

Insomnia can be treated by cutting down on caffeinated drinks, having milk at bedtime, not napping during the day, exercising early in the day, and discussing sleep-inducing medication with your doctor. (in some cases, discussing just about anything with your doctor might put you to sleep!)

Eating out

Ah... dining out. No cooking. No cleaning up. Delicious food. Pleasant company.

Don't we wish it was that simple? Dining out can present challenges to those with diabetes, especially when it comes to taking and timing the insulin injection, and measuring what's in that delicious plate (or plates) of food.

There are a few tricks to taking insulin at restaurants. If it doesn't bother you to take insulin in public, go right ahead and give your shot as you normally would. (Of course, if you usually give your shot in the buttocks, it may be wise to do so in the bathroom.)

However, if you're the type who feels uncomfortable about taking insulin in mixed company, you could simply excuse yourself and go to the rest room. Using a pre-filled insulin pen (no need to draw up insulin) might ease your discomfort.

Do NOT take your insulin before leaving for a restaurant. Wait until you are ready to be seated.

Timing the insulin depends on what your blood sugar is and whether or not food (bread, appetizers) will be available to you very soon after you are seated. Obviously, a high blood sugar means that you should take your insulin earlier than if it is in a normal range. If your blood sugar is within a good range and food will be available soon after you are seated, take your insulin when you are taken to your table. Do NOT take it before you leave home, because there may be a wait for a table. If the service at the restaurant is generally slow, you may want to wait until after you have placed your order to take your shot.

Now for that delicious meal. Ever wonder what makes it so delicious? Us too. About all we know for sure is that food eaten in restaurants tends to raise blood sugar more than similar types of food eaten at home. If you frequent fast food restaurants, there are a number of excellent booklets describing the carbohydrate, protein and fat content of many menu items. These booklets are available free of charge from B-D and Eli Lilly and Company.

When dining at sit-down restaurants, many people will count the grams of carbohydrate in the meal, and then add a 25% "restaurant factor". If your meal is high in protein or fat, you may need to make some of the adjustments described above in the section on Fat and Protein. Try these adjustment the next time you dine out and see how they work. If necessary, make further adjustments until your blood sugar levels look good several hours after dining.

Travel

Whether you travel often or just occasionally, being away from home can cause a host of problems with your blood sugar control. Anticipate that you will be sitting (i.e. inactive and not very insulin-sensitive) for long periods of time while you are in transit. If you change time zones or travel during off-peak hours, it would be to your benefit to be on an insulin pump or a multiple injection schedule for the sake of flexibility.

Food on airlines can unpredictable, not to mention scary at times. Some airlines offer "diabetic meals" upon request. While we all know that there is no real need for a "diabetic" meal, these meals can sometimes be much more tasty and nutritious than the usual airline fare. Whatever type of meal you choose, never take your insulin until you see the food coming down the aisle, and always carry some healthy snacks with you.

Drug/Alcohol Abuse

Most drugs and alcohol have indirect effects that may result in very high or low blood sugar levels. Drug addictions and alcohol abuse can cause people to miss meals, forget to take injections, or crave food. Alcohol can also render your liver incapable of releasing sugar into the bloodstream in response to hypoglycemia. If you drink, do so in moderation, and snack while you drink to prevent your blood sugar from going too low. Don't forget to count the carbohydrates in your alcoholic beverages!

Use of narcotics and other illicit drugs can easily kill you if you have diabetes. Talk to your doctor if you want to quit or just want more information.

Menstruation

During menstrual cycles, the body produces hormones that can raise and lower blood sugar levels. Many women find that their blood sugar levels are higher during the pre-menstrual cycle, and drop back down to normal levels after their period begins. Other women see different patterns entirely. If you notice unusually high or low blood sugar readings before, during or after your period, talk to your doctor about developing a set of strategies for these times of the month.

For example, you may need to raise your insulin doses by 20% a week before you are due for your period, and then return to normal insulin doses when your period begins.

Monitoring mistakes

If the blood glucose meter you are using is not working correctly, or if you are not using it properly, the results can be very misleading. Common errors to watch out for include:

Meter Problem	Your Solution
Outdated strips	Check the expiration date before opening a box or vial or strips.
Using strips that have been exposed to heat or humidity.	Keep your strips sealed in their packaging and away from extreme temperatures. Do not leave strips in car!
Blood or dirt inside machine.	Clean your meter as described in owner's manual
Insufficient blood on the test strip. (#1 reason for incorrect readings!)	Obtain a large, hanging drop of blood before placing the blood on the strip.

If you want to confirm the accuracy of your meter, compare the result to a laboratory blood report. Don't try comparing the results on your meter to the results on another meter, because the other meter may be incorrect. Test your blood at the same time your doctor draws blood from your arm, and note the result. The laboratory reading will probably be 10-15% higher simply because of the way the lab does the measurement. If the lab's number and your meter's number differ by more than 25%, you might consider purchasing a new meter.

Other medications

Certain medications, especially "steroidal" medications such as cortisone and prednisone (Deltasone) can impair insulin's ability to lower blood sugar. These types of drugs are commonly used to treat asthma, arthritis, emphysema and muscle/joint disorders. When taking a steroidal medication, monitor your blood sugar carefully. If you see a rise in your blood sugar, discuss it with your doctor; it may be necessary to increase your insulin dose. Temporary changes in the dosage of steroidal medications can also lead to higher-than-normal blood sugar levels. People who control their diabetes without pills or insulin may find that they need them, at least temporarily, while taking steroidal medications.

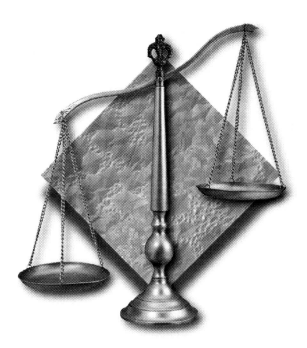

Chapter 14: Hypoglycemia

Hypoglycemia means low blood sugar (readings below 70 mg/dl). Unlike high blood sugar, which carries long-term risks, low blood sugar is dangerous the moment it happens. It can cause you to fall, get into an accident, lose control of your senses or lose consciousness. If not treated quickly, it can cause you to have seizures, go into a coma, or even die. Hypoglycemia is serious stuff that requires serious and immediate action. It can be caused by a variety of factors, but generally is due to a severe imbalance: The factors lowering your blood sugar far outweigh the factors raising it (see next page).

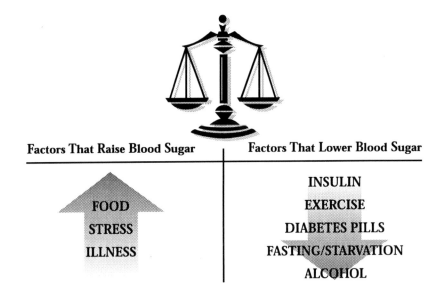

Factors That Raise Blood Sugar	Factors That Lower Blood Sugar
FOOD	INSULIN
STRESS	EXERCISE
ILLNESS	DIABETES PILLS
	FASTING/STARVATION
	ALCOHOL

Common causes of low blood sugar

The most common causes of low blood sugar are either too little food or too much exercise in relation to the amount of insulin or medication that was taken. Anyone taking insulin can get low blood sugar if they are not careful to match their insulin dose to their carbohydrate intake and physical activities. Timing is also important for those who take insulin; meals must be consumed prior to the peak action time of the insulin. That means that meals must be eaten 3-5 hours after taking NPH or Lente insulin; 1/2 to 1 hour after taking regular insulin, and 0-15 minutes after taking Humalog.

Those taking diabetes pills are susceptible to low blood sugar as well. Sulfonylureas (OHAs) can cause low blood sugar if food is not eaten in the proper amounts and at the proper times, and if exercise is excessive. Metformin and Precose, when taken without an OHA or insulin, will not cause low blood sugar.

Other causes of low blood sugar include:

- Very hot or humid conditions, since this speeds the absorption and action of insulin.

- Hypothyroidism (under-active thyroid gland), since this increases sensitivity to insulin and OHAs.

- Kidney disease, since it takes longer for certain OHAs to be eliminated from the body. If you have kidney disease and are taking an older drug such as chlorpropamide (Diabinese), you run a high risk of low blood sugar.

- Injecting insulin into a site that will be exercised soon afterward, since this speeds the absorption and action of the insulin.

- Taking an incorrect dose of insulin, or mixing up the bottles.

- Overtreating a high blood sugar after a meal by taking an additional dose of insulin before the pre-meal dose has worked completely (Humalog: 3-5 hours; regular: 5-7 hours; NPH/Lente: 12-16 hours).

- Excessive alcohol consumption, because it keeps the liver from releasing sugar into the bloodstream the way it normally does, and may cause you to forget to have your usual meals or snacks.

- Changes of environment (new job, new house, starting school) because the brain is working overtime to become acclimated to the new surroundings, and burns much more energy than usual.

- Digestive disorders such as gastroparesis, in which food is digested very slowly or carbohydrate absorption is impaired.

- Beginning menstruation, since abrupt hormonal changes may trigger a rapid decline in blood sugar levels.

Symptoms and treatment of low blood sugar

Low blood sugar comes in three stages: mild, moderate, and severe. You might call them "the good, the bad, and the ugly." Mild hypoglycemia is good because the physical symptoms give you a chance to raise your blood sugar before your thinking becomes impaired. Moderate hypoglycemia is bad because your mental functions have become impaired, and you may have trouble making important decisions. Severe hypoglycemia is ugly because you have lost the ability to help yourself, and will need outside assistance just to regain consciousness.

Below is a summary of the symptoms and proper treatment for each stage of hypoglycemia:

	SYMPTOMS	TREATMENT*
Mild Hypoglycemia • Blood sugar 50 - 70	"Physical" symptoms only: • Shaking/trembling • Sweating • Weakness • Pallor • Pounding heart	10-15 grams of simple sugar, such as: • 1/2 cup regular soda (not diet) • 1/2 cup orange juice • 2-3 B-D glucose tablets • 3-4 Can-Am Dex Tabs • 6-8 lifesavers
Moderate Hypoglycemia • Blood sugar 35 -50	"Brain and Nerve" symptoms, with or without physical symptoms • Confusion • Slurred Speech • Poor coordination. • Disorientation • Short attention span • Mood change	• 15-30 grams of simple sugar (double the amounts given above)
Severe Hypoglycemia • Blood sugar usually less than 35	Inability to think and act in order to treat low blood sugar. • Man be unconscious • Having a seizure • Violent or "out of control" • Comatose	• Glucagon injection, or sugary gel (ICN InstaGlucose, or cake gel) if unconscious and glucagon is not available. • Follow up with 15 grams of ordinary carbohydrate.

* Re-check your blood sugar in 15 minutes and take another 15 grams of simple sugar if it is still below 70. If the next meal is more than 1/2 hour away, follow the simple sugar with a high-protein snack such as cheese, peanut butter or milk.

Foods high in fat, such as chocolate or potato chips, are not good choices for treating low blood sugar because the fat slows the absorption of sugar into the bloodstream. Foods high in fiber, such as whole fruits and vegetables, may have a similar effect.

Check before you treat

It may seem ridiculous, but it is possible to have symptoms of low blood sugar without actually having low blood sugar.

For example, you could feel low when your blood sugar is very high. High blood sugar triggers similar symptoms as low blood sugar (edginess, weakness, hunger). That's why you should always check your blood to confirm that your sugar is actually low before treating it as such. After all, if your blood sugar is 280 and you take 15 grams of simple carbohydrate thinking that it is low, it could go up to 350, and the symptoms could become worse.

If your control has been poor for quite some time and you suddenly tighten your control, you may start to experience low blood sugar even if the readings are 80 and above.

Also, a sudden drop in blood sugar can trigger symptoms of hypoglycemia. Going from 300 down to 150 in an hour may make you feel low without actually being low.

Of course, if you suspect that your blood sugar is low but are not able to check it, go ahead and treat it. It is always better to treat it than to risk severe hypoglycemia.

Glucagon

When the blood sugar is severely low, it is possible to lose consciousness. At this point, it would be dangerous to have someone try to give you sugar by mouth. If you don't bite their fingers off, chances are you will choke on whatever is being fed to you. This is a job for glucagon!

Glucagon is a hormone given by injection that does just the opposite of insulin - it raises blood sugar by forcing the liver to release lots of sugar into the bloodstream. A single injection of glucagon will only raise the blood sugar about 50 points, which is just enough to allow you to regain consciousness and be aware enough to treat the situation with an additional 15 grams of simple carbohydrate.

Everyone who takes insulin or an OHA (oral hypoglycemic agent) should have glucagon on hand at all times. If you spend a great deal of time away from home (at the office, for example), it would be a good idea to keep an extra kit there as well. More importantly, someone close to you should be instructed on when and how to give the glucagon injection. Remember, it should only be used if you are unconscious or unable to take sugar by mouth. If your partner is not sure that your blood sugar is low, they should prick your finger and check your blood sugar before giving glucagon.

Glucagon is available by prescription only. Each kit comes with a syringe filled with liquid, and a vial containing the glucagon hormone in a powdery pill form. The hormone will lose its potency over time, so it will be necessary to purchase a fresh kit every year or so. Check the expiration date to see when your kit should be replaced.

Giving an injection of glucagon is a simple 4-step procedure:

1) Inject the fluid contained in the syringe into the vial.

2) Mix the vial until the glucagon "pill" is completely dissolved.

3) Draw the solution back into the syringe. Draw up to the 1.0 mark for adults; the .5 mark for school-age children; the .25 mark for infants and very small children.

4) Insert the needle into the buttocks, and inject the full amount. A small amount of blood may appear. This is perfectly normal and should not be a cause for concern. Occasionally, vomiting will occur. Simply turn the person on his/her side to prevent choking.

After giving glucagon, wait about 15-20 minutes. If the person has not regained consciousness, a 2nd injection with another glucagon kit may be given. If consciousness is not regained after two injections, or if a second kit is not available, call 911.

Note: If a person has low blood sugar and has been drinking alcohol, glucagon will probably not work (alcohol opposes the action of glucagon). In this event, glucose must be given intravenously, so 911 should be called.

As described in the symptoms/treatment chart earlier in the chapter, it may be possible to use a sugary gel such as cake icing or InstaGlucose if glucagon is not available. Fluids and solids can cause choking, but gel placed inside the cheek can be absorbed directly through the lining of the mouth and into the bloodstream, and poses little choking risk. Be sure that the victim is lying on his/her side when gel is given.

Too much of a good thing

One of the most common mistakes made by people with low blood sugar is overtreating it with too much food (See Chapter 13: Sources of Uncontrolled Diabetes, Overtreatment of Lows). It is certainly understandable for a person to want to eat a lot when the blood sugar is low. You feel weak and very hungry, and you know that food will make the symptoms go away. You may even think that this is your "golden opportunity" to indulge on sweets.

This is where discipline separates the tough guys from the wannabees. EATING TOO MUCH <u>WILL</u> LEAD TO HIGH BLOOD SUGAR IN THE NEXT COUPLE OF HOURS. Knowing that, you can work up strategies to keep yourself from overtreating low blood sugar. Have a specific treatment ready for whenever you get low. Perhaps it could be glucose tablets. Or perhaps it could be pre-measured containers of juice. Whatever you choose, make sure that it is <u>all</u> you use. Keep it out of the kitchen so you won't be tempted by everything else in the refrigerator. If necessary, plan to occupy yourself while waiting for your blood sugar to come up by reading a magazine, watching TV, talking to someone, or even playing solitaire. It may take up to half an hour for the symptoms to disappear completely, so be patient — you don't need two problems for the price of one. Treat hypoglycemia appropriately and be done with it.

Preventing the lows

Now we get to the good stuff. In virtually all instances, low blood sugar can be prevented through discipline and common sense. The most common causes of low blood sugar are a delay in a meal, too small a meal to cover the amount of insulin taken, and unexpected activity. By making sure to eat at consistent times and in consistent amounts, and snacking when you are more physically active than usual, you can avoid low blood sugar in most cases. If you know that a meal will be delayed or are not sure of the contents of a meal, plan to snack ahead of time to "carry you over" until you have a chance for a full meal.

Here are some other suggestions from people with diabetes who have learned to avoid low blood sugar:

1) Check your blood sugar often. Besides providing you and your doctor with valuable information for adjusting your insulin and medications, monitoring will help warn you of an upcoming low blood sugar. For example, if you take insulin and have a reading of <100 at bedtime, you can snack to avoid low blood sugar during the night.

2) Keep you doctor up to date on all the drugs (prescription and over-the-counter) that you are taking. Certain drugs may interact and put you at risk for hypoglycemia. For example, some of the older OHAs can react with aspirin and become more potent.

3) If you are taking one of the older drugs for treating diabetes (see chapter 4), talk to your doctor about switching to one of the newer drugs. The more recent medications carry a much lower risk of hypoglycemia.

4) At the first sign of low blood sugar, treat it. Don't wait a single minute. The symptoms will become worse, and if it drops low enough, you may not be able to think clearly enough to treat it appropriately.

5) Plan for possible emergencies. Keep packaged carbohydrates in your car in case of a delay. Keep food at work in case lunch is delayed or you are forced to work late. Keep glucose tablets with you at all times in case you are detained somewhere and cannot make it home for your regular mealtime. For example, many people who use mass transit (buses, subways, etc.) are delayed when the weather is bad. Having carbohydrates with you can tide you over until you can get home.

6) If you plan to go on a low-calorie diet or start an exercise program, talk to your doctor about reducing your dosage of insulin or OHA.

7) If you plan to exercise soon after a meal, inject your insulin into a part of the body that will not be very active. For example, if you plan to walk, jog or ride a bike, inject your insulin into your abdomen.

8) When the weather gets hot, you may need to reduce your dose of insulin. Hot weather causes the blood vessels in the skin to dilate, which leads to faster insulin absorption and action.

9) Avoid mixing up your insulin bottles by labeling one with tape or by keeping one bottle in its original box.

10) If you accidentally take too much insulin, be sure to check your blood sugar and eat extra food for the next four hours (if too much regular or Humalog was injected), or 8 hours (if too much NPH or Lente was injected).

11) Learn how exercise affects your blood sugar by monitoring before and after a workout. If your blood sugar drops by 50 points it should be at least 130 before you start, or you risk going too low. Extra snacking may be necessary before exercising.

12) Treat any extra physical activity (mowing the lawn, housework, shopping, etc.) as a factor that lowers your blood sugar. You may not be getting the same benefits as a true exercise session, but your blood sugar can go down with any increase in activity. Prepare to snack and check your blood sugar more often than usual.

13) If you forget to take your insulin and wind up taking it much later than usual, take only 1/2 or 2/3 of the full dose. Otherwise, it will overlap with your next injection and may cause low blood sugar later in the day or night.

14) Be on the lookout for delayed hypoglycemia after a particularly strenuous workout. This type of low blood sugar can occur 12-24 hours after exercise. Check your blood sugar a little more frequently following a tough workout, and be prepared to snack and possibly reduce your post-exercise insulin dose the next time around.

15) Set realistic blood sugar targets. Aiming for readings of 70 to 120 before meals may be too tight, especially if you are taking insulin. It simply doesn't leave any margin for error. Aiming for readings of 80 to 150 or 100 to 180 may be more realistic, and certainly allows some margin for error before you become hypoglycemic.

Pattern adjustments for low blood sugar

Based on your experiences, it is easy to come up with a plan to prevent low blood sugar in the future. Any consistent pattern of low blood sugar may indicate a need to change some aspect of your diabetes therapy:

If you are getting low blood sugar...	Try these adjustments
Before breakfast	Reduce your overnight long-acting insulin -or- Take you nighttime insulin later in the evening -or- Have a larger bedtime snack -or- Add protein to the bedtime snack
Mid-Morning/Before lunch	Increase the size of your breakfast -or- Snack at mid-morning -or- Reduce your morning R or Humalog
Afternoon/Before Dinner	Increase the size of your lunch -or- Snack in the afternoon -or- Reduce morning NPH or Lente
Evening/Before Bedtime	Increase the size of your dinner -or- Reduce your dinnertime R or Humalog

Other general adjustments that can be made for consistently low readings are: (1) changing the composition of your meals and (2) switching to a more rapid-acting insulin.

Adding some protein to a meal will delay the absorption of the carbo-hydrates into the bloodstream, so your blood sugar will rise steadily for a longer period of time. This may prevent low blood sugar before the next meal.

Likewise, switching to a faster-acting insulin (human insulin instead of beef/pork insulin; Humalog instead of Regular; NPH instead of

Lente) will move the peak time of the insulin closer to the time you are eating. That way, the insulin will not be peaking several hours after a meal, and is less likely to cause low blood sugar.

Hypoglycemic Unawareness

Having being married for many years, it is easy to start taking things for granted. We don't listen as closely, aren't quite as sensitive, and may learn to "tune out" our partner. Unless a major crisis arises, communication can be virtually non-existent. Call it "spousal unawareness."

After having had diabetes for many years, most people with diabetes lose the early warning signs of hypoglycemia: the shaking, sweating, paleness and rapid heartbeat. In fact, many people don't know they have a low blood sugar until the level drops to the 50s, 40s or 30s. By that time, the most noticeable symptoms are due to impaired thought processes - confusion, poor coordination, slurred speech, and so on. This is called "hypoglycemic unawareness." The body has lost its ability to produce adrenaline in response to mild hypoglycemia. Symptoms are not detected until the brain is deprived of its only energy source: sugar.

DRIVERS WARNING:

Before operating a motor vehicle or any heavy machinery, check you blood sugar. Low blood sugar can impair you ability to operate a vehicle safely, and can cause damage to equipment or harm to yourself and other people.

People with hypoglycemic unawareness are at a major risk to have accidents, make poor decisions and lose consciousness due to severe hypoglycemia. For these folks, it is very important to check the blood sugar several times a day, eat at regular intervals, and set blood sugar targets that are not too "tight" — perhaps 100-200 before meals. In other words, leave a little margin for error to reduce the risk of hypoglycemia in the first place.

Is hypoglycemic unawareness reversible? Yes, but it takes a conscious effort to avoid low blood sugar entirely for several weeks or months. In many cases, some of the early warning signs of hypoglycemia return after a person has gone for a while without any low blood sugars.

Smogyi (rebound) effect

Low blood sugar in the middle of the night while you sleep is particularly dangerous since you are not awake to notice the symptoms or treat it. In fact, you could wake up with perfectly normal, or even high, blood sugar readings after having hypoglycemia while you sleep. This is called a "rebound" or "Smogyi" effect (after the doctor who discovered it). When your blood sugar goes a little bit low, the liver starts to slowly release sugar into the bloodstream. After a few hours, the blood sugar might return to normal, or even go above normal.

The only way to find out if you are going too low and then rebounding during the night is by doing an occasional 3 a.m. blood sugar check. Let's look at two examples:

Steve goes to sleep with a blood sugar of 130. He checks at 3 a.m. and his reading is 55. He has a small snack and wakes up in the morning with a blood sugar of 190. He is definitely dropping and then rebounding, so he either needs to reduce his nighttime insulin or have a larger bedtime snack.

Stan, on the other hand, goes to bed with a blood sugar of 130. At 3 a.m. he is 160; by morning he is up to 190. Stan and Steve both started and finished the night with the same blood sugar levels.

However, where Steve's problem was a low in the middle of the night, Stan is clearly not taking enough insulin to keep his blood sugar stable through the night. Amazing what you can learn from a little bit of monitoring!

Key Point:

Hypoglycemia, or low blood sugar, occurs when the factors lowering the blood sugar exceed the factors raising it. Through discipline and common sense, low blood sugar can be properly treated as well as prevented.

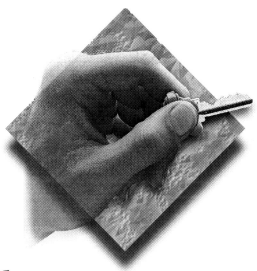

Chapter 15:

Dealing with Hyperglycemia, Illness and Infection

Hyperglycemia means high blood sugar. For a person without diabetes, any blood sugar reading over 140 would be considered hyperglycemia. For those with diabetes, hyperglycemia takes on a whole new meaning. If you are attempting to keep tight, intensive control of your blood sugars, you might consider any reading over 180 to be hyperglycemia. If your control is still relatively "loose", 240 and up might represent hyperglycemia. In any case, one thing we can all agree on is this: **Blood sugars that are higher than you want or expect represent hyperglycemia.**

The problem with hyperglycemia is that it makes you feel like a slug in the short term, and increases your risk for complications in the long term. High blood sugar makes people feel tired, weak, hungry and slow. Sugar in the blood also sticks to everything in sight - proteins, muscles, blood vessel walls and so on - causing long-term damage to the eyes, kidneys, nerves and large blood vessels leading to the brain, heart and legs. Any way you look at it, hyperglycemia is nasty and should not be put up with.

Causes of hyperglycemia

Hyperglycemia is caused by an imbalance between the factors that raise and lower blood sugar. In other words, you may have eaten too much food (carbohydrate, to be exact), not taken enough medication or insulin, been under a great deal of stress, or are not getting enough exercise. If you have Type-II diabetes, weight gain will make your insulin less effective, so you may see your blood sugar levels rise over time. A traumatic experience such as a car accident, an argument with a loved one, being victimized by crime, or suffering a broken bone can also cause high blood sugar due to the release of stress hormones.

When your blood sugar is running high, your choices are simple. You could do nothing about it and continue to feel like a slug and risk damage to your eyes, kidneys, nerves, feet and heart. Or you could take action to get your blood sugar back into balance. This could include:

• <u>Lowering your carbohydrate intake</u>. For example, you could replace some of your starchy foods with green vegetables. Sugary beverages and juices could be replaced with sugar-free drinks. Portion sizes of cereals, pastas, rice and bread products could be reduced by a third or half.

- <u>Getting more exercise</u>. Look for every opportunity to walk and be more physically active throughout the day.

- <u>Losing weight</u>. Reducing calorie intake (by limiting portion sizes and minimizing fats in your diet) in conjunction with increasing physical activity should produce safe, gradual weight loss and improvements in your insulin sensitivity and blood sugar control.

- <u>Managing stress</u>. Stress management techniques such as yoga, progressive relaxation, meditation, and even cardiovascular exercise can reduce the impact of stress on your blood sugar levels.

- <u>Taking more medication or insulin</u>. Increasing your dosage of insulin is a sure-fire way to lower your blood sugar levels. But don't forget, increasing your dosage of OHA or insulin may cause you to gain weight, which could be counterproductive to your long-term health.

The ill effects of illness and infection

Infections are common in people with diabetes, especially when the blood sugar is high. White blood cells which fight infection do not work well when blood sugar is high, so bacteria has a chance to grow and spread. In turn, infection causes the body to produce stress hormones which drive the blood sugar even higher and make insulin less effective. This makes the infection even worse, so the cycle keeps going (see next below).

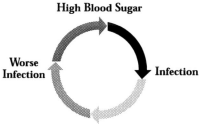

Infection can occur in a variety of ways. You could have a respiratory infection (bronchitis, pneumonia); vaginal or urinary tract infection; an open wound infection (especially on the feet); or a viral infection (complete with low grade fever, aches and pains, vomiting or diarrhea).

When you have an infection, the following symptoms are common. Be on the lookout for them because they may help you detect an infection and treat it before it becomes very serious:

Symptoms of infection

- High blood sugar through most of the day and night.

- Nausea (possibly with diarrhea or vomiting)

- Fever

- Dehydration; a feeling of dryness

- Areas of skin that look red or swollen, feel warm, or have pus.

Diabetes care on "sick days"

It is VERY IMPORTANT to take care of your diabetes when you get sick. Not because high sugars may affect your HbA1c or because low sugars might force you to eat even if you are not hungry. Those are the least of your problems. The things to worry about are dehydration and diabetic ketoacidosis - a life-threatening condition caused by very high blood sugar and not having enough insulin during illness. Both will land you in the emergency room with a bunch of tubes and needles sticking out of you. So, presented here, for your sick-day entertainment, is a checklist of MUST-DO's and DON'T-YOU-DARE-DO's for managing diabetes when you are ill:

MUST DO'S

• <u>Call your doctor</u> at the first sign of illness or infection (see symptoms of infection above). Keep in touch with your doctor frequently during your illness.

• <u>Take your insulin</u> (or diabetes medication), even if you are not eating as much as usual. If you don't normally take insulin, you may need to take some now. If you already take insulin, an additional amount may be required. This extra insulin is called a "sick day booster." The body's insulin needs go up when we are sick because insulin does not work as well during illness, and extra help is needed to lower the blood sugar. Below are guidelines for taking a sick day booster:

BOOSTER GUIDELINES

• Use only fast-acting insulin for a booster. Maintain usual doses of intermediate and long-acting insulin, and add the booster to your usual insulin doses.

• Boosters should be given prior to meals, and after checking blood sugar and urine ketones.

• If you are sick and have high blood sugar with no ketones in your urine, add 10% of your total daily dose as a booster.

• If you are sick and have high blood sugar with ketones in your urine, add 20% of your total daily dose as a booster.

• For example, if you normally take a grand total of 40 units of insulin a day, you would add 10% (4 units) of fast-acting insulin to your usual pre-meal insulin doses if you don't have ketones; 20% (8 units) if you do have ketones.

• <u>Set up a sliding scale</u>. No, you won't be taking your bathroom scale to the park. A sliding scale means that you adjust your insulin dose based on how high your blood sugar is. It is usually a good idea to take fast-acting insulin every 4-6 hours. If you already take insulin, you could simply add this to your usual dosage. For example, the following sliding scale is used by people who normally take a total of 60-75 units of insulin a day (people who take less insulin will need less in their sliding scale to cover high blood sugar; those who take more insulin will require larger sliding scale doses):

SLIDING SCALE	
If blood sugar is ...	**Take this much extra fast-acting insulin***
Less than 200	0 units
200 - 250	4 units
250 - 300	8 units
300 - 400	12 units
over 400	18 units

* Note: If your blood sugar remains high despite taking sliding scale insulin, try increasing the sliding scale by 50%. Instead of 4 units, take 6. Instead of 8 units, take 12, and so on.

• <u>Drink plenty of liquids</u>. By plenty, you should be having at least one cup (8 ounces) of fluid every hour. As you know, high blood sugar causes you to urinate more, whether or not your body is dehydrated to begin with. If you are vomiting or have diarrhea, you may be losing fluids by the bucket. To replace the lost fluids, have decaffeinated, clear, sugar-free beverages, water or Jello. If you are having trouble keeping solid food down, try alternating sugar-free fluids with fluids that contain about 15 grams of carbohydrate every other hour. For example, one hour you could have diet 7-up; the next hour you could have 8 oz. Gatorade or 4 oz. regular 7-Up or 8 oz. diluted juice (half juice, half water).

KETONES AND KETOACIDOSIS

Ketones are an end product of fat burning, similar to smoke that comes from burning coal. When sugar is burned along with fat, the ketones get burned up as well, like wind clearing smoke away. If not enough sugar is getting into the cells (due to a lack of insulin), ketones can build up. Ketones are acid-like chemicals that can damage the body. If too many ketones reach the bloodstream, it can lead to a life-threatening condition called diabetic ketoacidosis (DKA).

• <u>Monitor Often</u>. If you are not doing it already, check your blood sugar every 4-6 hours (before every meal and at bedtime) when you are sick. If you are used to adjusting your insulin dose based on your pre-meal blood sugar, go ahead and do so, and don't forget to add your "booster dose". Be sure to write down your blood sugars so that you can keep your doctor informed. If your blood sugar is higher than usual, be sure to check your urine for ketones. The presence of ketones means that your body is not getting enough insulin. A 20% "booster dose" will be needed if you have ketones in your urine. Ketostix can be obtained from your pharmacy, either in a vial or foil-wrapped form (Miles Diagnostics - see Appendix B).

• <u>Get plenty of rest</u>. Your body needs all its energy to fight the infection and help you get better.

- <u>Check your temperature regularly.</u> If it is above normal (98.6), report the result to your doctor immediately. Fever does not always occur with infection, but if you have a fever, it usually means that an infection exists somewhere in your body.

- <u>Keep a fresh bottle of fast-acting insulin in your refrigerator</u>, even if you don't normally use it. When you are sick, you may need to start using fast-acting insulin to get your blood sugar levels under control.

- <u>Get a flu vaccine every year.</u> While you're at it, make sure that you are up-to-date on all of your vaccinations, including the vaccine for pneumonia (needed every 5 - 10 years).

DON'T YOU DARE DO'S

- <u>Never stop taking your insulin or diabetes medication when you are sick.</u> Even if you don't have much of an appetite or can't keep food down, your stress hormones are still causing your liver to dump a ton of sugar into your blood stream. If you are vomiting, you are also losing a great deal of fluids, which can lower your blood volume and cause your blood sugar level to go up. Without insulin, your blood sugar will go much higher and your cells will starve for energy. If your cells cannot burn sugar for fuel, you will start producing ketones, a harmful substance that can damage your body and put you into a coma.

- <u>Do not rely on your thirst sensation to tell you when to drink.</u> When you are sick, you are likely to be less thirsty than usual, especially if your stomach is upset. You need more fluids when you are sick due to extra urination and dehydration caused by fever and infection. As described above, drink at least a cup of fluids every waking hour, whether you are thirsty or not.

- <u>Put off exercise.</u> Remember, your body needs its energy to fight the infection. In addition to using up precious energy, exercising while you are sick is likely to drive your blood sugar higher, cause greater ketone production, and dehydrate your body further.

"Sick happens": A heavy toll

Basic, seasonal colds and mild infections can occur in just about anybody. But every year, thousands of people with diabetes are hospitalized; some lose limbs, and some die when simple, treatable illnesses become much more serious problems such as severe dehydration, diabetic ketoacidosis, or widespread infection. By keeping your blood sugar well-controlled, watching for the early signs of infection, and following the sick-day do's and don'ts listed above, you can avoid these problems and keep a short-term illness in the short-term.

> **Key Point:**
> **Always call your doctor, drink plenty of fluids, and take your insulin or diabetes medication when you are sick.**

Section IV

Living With Diabetes: Real Solutions for Real-Life Challenges

Like the absent-minded professor who isn't smart enough to come in out of the rain, living well with diabetes takes more than just a "textbook" approach. Up to now, most of the information presented has been based on numbers, science, and predictable outcomes in a perfect world. But this is real life!!! It's a place where Murphy's Law rules, and S*!# Happens. To ignore real life situations would do you a great disservice. This section will present and (hopefully) prepare you for some of the common issues that people with diabetes must contend with in the real world.

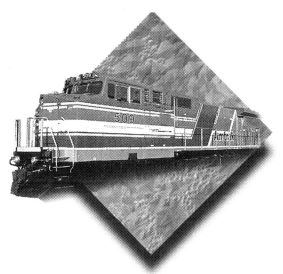

Chapter 16:

How to Get Off Insulin or Medication (the weight loss factor)

Hope the drug companies don't find out about this chapter! If you have Type-II diabetes and are a few pounds overweight, chances are very good that you can get off insulin or medication for your diabetes.

THE RUNAWAY TRAIN OF DIABETIC WEIGHT GAIN

The "miracle cure" for Type-II diabetes can be summed up in two words: <u>Healthy</u> <u>Livin'</u> — the kind that brings about moderate and permanent weight loss. You see, obesity makes insulin lose most of its blood sugar-lowering ability. Overweight people have to take (or make) large amounts of insulin to keep the blood sugar level down.

Unfortunately, insulin also increases your appetite and leads to weight gain, which in turn makes your insulin even less effective and forces your dosage to increase.

Whenever you try to cut down your food intake, the insulin makes you want to eat everything in sight. This is especially true when the insulin is peaking, 2-4 hours after taking Regular insulin or 4-8 hours after taking NPH or Lente insulin. And all that extra eating, of course, causes even more weight gain, not to mention frustration. It's like a runaway train rolling down a mountain, getting faster and more dangerous with every roll.

APPLYING THE BRAKES

The good news is that the runaway train of diabetic weight gain can be stopped. It is possible to lose weight and reduce your need for insulin or diabetes pills, but it will take a strong effort on your part. The choice is yours: Continue rolling downhill toward a life of poor health and disability, or take a stand now and turn this train around. The rewards are plentiful — better appearance, more energy and zest for life, reduced dependency on shots and medication, and a sharply reduced risk of long-term diabetic complications.

So let's get going. Weight loss is a serious matter that requires planning and commitment. Here are our "top 10" recommendations to help make it work for you:

Weight Loss Trick #1:

Write down realistic goals.

Writing down your goals and putting them up in a prominent place like your refrigerator or bathroom mirror helps refresh your commitment every day. A realistic goal may be to lose 20 pounds at a time. 20 pounds is usually enough to improve the effectiveness of your insulin, resulting in improved blood sugar levels. It's a well-deserved reward for a job well done.

After losing 20 pounds, work on maintaining your weight for 2-3 months, making sure not to gain any of the weight back. Limit your weigh-ins to once weekly so as not to become overly concerned with temporary water-weight gain or loss. Once your weight has stabilized, your metabolism will also adjust. Then, it is time to work on the next 10, or 15 or 20 pounds, depending on your weight loss needs.

Weight Loss Trick #2:

Exercise Is A MUST!

As a soaking sailor once said, "Trying to lose weight without exercise is like trying to bail out a sinking ship with a spoon."

Exercise, with or without weight loss, can play a vital role in improving the power of your body's own insulin. Imagine insulin as keys, going around to the cells of your body and opening doors to allow sugar to enter. In a body that doesn't exercise, the keys move very slowly from door to door, so only a small amount of sugar is leaving the bloodstream and entering the cells. However, in a body that exercises regularly, the keys become "super-charged". They zip around from door to door and cell to cell, opening everything in sight.

As a result, blood sugar levels are lower, and our cells have plenty of fuel to burn.

Why is exercise so important when we are trying to lose weight? Several reasons. But first, let's look at the weight loss equation (Don't panic! I promise there won't be any math.)

CALORIES OUT - CALORIES IN = WEIGHT LOSS CALORIES

In other words, burn more calories than you eat, and you will lose weight. We know how to cut the "calories in": eat less food, especially high-calorie fatty foods. But how do we increase the "calories out"? By exercising! A brisk 45 minute walk can help you burn 200 extra calories each day. Since it takes a 3500 calorie deficit to lose one pound of fat, you can easily lose a pound of fat a week by eliminating or substituting high-fat foods with low-fat foods and walking each day. Trying to lose more than 1-2 pounds of fat a week is unrealistic and not conducive to permanent weight loss.

All you exercise haters are probably doing the math and saying, "what if I just cut more calories from my diet? Then would I need to exercise?"

'Fraid so, pardner. Because of an ornery critter called "metabolism". To understand the role of metabolism, lets look at what is happening to Native Americans.

Hundreds of years ago, the Indians were able to survive famine because their bodies would conserve fuel — burning fewer calories while doing the same amount of work — when food was scarce. Even though they ate less, they could still survive because their metabolism slowed down.

The same thing happens when we cut our calorie intake. Our bodies perceive this to be a famine situation, and we start to burn fewer calories when doing the same amount of work. Sounds like our "calories out" are starting to suffer, doesn't it? It's the ultimate "catch 22": You try to lose weight, so your body slows down to keep you from losing weight. That's why many people gain back more weight after they stop dieting — they return to their old level of "calories in", but their "calories out" are lower than before.

Exercise to the rescue! Aerobic exercises like walking, swimming and cycling burn lots of calories to help keep our "calories out" high. And strength training exercise — the kind that builds and tones muscles — can actually increase metabolism by giving us more energy-burning muscle tissue than we had before.

As an added bonus, exercise will help keep your spirits up while bringing your weight down. It can also keep you occupied (i.e. not snacking) while watching TV. Or better yet, get you away from the tube entirely!

Weight Loss Trick #3:

Control Your Blood Sugar

Get your morning blood sugar under 150 before starting your weight loss program.

Last spring, a woman went into her doctor's office with a look of amazement on her face. "Doctor, look at this," she said. She proceeded to pull out her blood glucose logbook. It looked like most other logbooks — sloppy, tattered, and smeared with blood.

"Doctor, I figured out why I have trouble losing weight. I get hungry whenever my blood sugar goes up!"

Indeed, she was right. Her records clearly showed that she ate more whenever her blood sugar was over 150. In fact, many people with diabetes have found that high blood sugar increases the appetite. That's why it is so important for you and your doctor to make whatever adjustments are necessary to get your fasting (pre-breakfast) blood sugar down under 150 before starting your weight loss program.

Now you're probably saying, "Hold on! I thought this chapter was all about getting off insulin and medication. Now you want me to take more?"

As successful business people know, sometimes you have to spend money to make money. Think of this initial dosage increase as a wise investment towards your long-term weight loss and independence from pills and insulin.

As we discussed earlier, you will start seeing your blood sugar come down as your weight comes down. When you start seeing readings below 100, or if you experience hypoglycemia (low blood sugar), throw your hands in the air and yell HALLELUJAH! It's time to talk dosage reduction.

Usually, cutting the medication dose by 1/2-3/4 or the insulin dose by 10-20% will bring the fasting blood sugar back to the 140-150 range. Continue exercising and reducing your calorie intake, and your blood sugar will begin dropping again. Once again, cut the dose and monitor your blood sugar frequently.

Weight Loss Trick #4:

Don't Skip Meals.

Sorry, brunch lovers. It is better to eat three meals a day than just two. Three evenly-spaced meals maximize the calories your body burns digesting food. In other words, you will burn more if you have a normal breakfast and lunch than if you skip breakfast or lunch and have a large supper. Modest, frequent meals will also help you to control your blood sugar better than one or two large meals.

Weight Loss Trick #5:

Become "Food Smart"

Life is getting busier. Most of us don't have time to prepare fresh meals from scratch anymore. With literally thousands of processed and "fast" foods for us to choose from, the smart dieter must learn how to read labels and make smart choices.

A) Count calories. When it comes to weight loss, calories are the only things that really matter. That statement is so important, Let's repeat it. <u>When it comes to weight loss, calories are the only things that really matter</u>. And every calorie counts equally — whether it comes from fat (9 calories per gram), alcohol (6 calories per gram), protein (4 calories per gram) or carbohydrate (4 calories per gram). Of course, substituting a gram of fat with a gram of protein or carbohydrate will reduce your total calorie intake. For example, a 4-ounce serving of low-fat frozen yogurt contains about 100 calories, while 4 ounces of ice cream contains about 150. Same size portions — but one has more carbohydrate, the other more fat.

Just don't get the idea that something will help you lose weight just because it is low in fat. If it contains carbohydrate, protein or alcohol, it still has calories, and it can still cause weight gain if eaten in large quantities.

B) Select low-calorie snacks. Instead of chips, nuts, cookies and candy, choose pretzels, low-fat popcorn, yogurt, or fresh fruits/vegetables.

C) Avoid liquid calories, such as those found in beverages sweetened with sugar. A single can of regular soda contains anywhere from 120 to 180 calories. A can of diet soda usually contains none. Choose sugar free items whenever possible — if not for diabetes control, then to help with weight loss.

D) Pay attention to portion sizes. Here is an example: A few years ago, there was a college professor who couldn't figure out why his blood sugar went up so high after breakfast. "All I'm having is a cup of cereal, half a cup of milk, and a piece of toast," he insisted. When we had him prepare and then measure his typical breakfast, he found that he was actually having almost two cups of cereal and a full cup of milk with his toast. What's more, he wasn't accounting for the jelly spread he put on his toast. What this means is that you could be having almost twice as many calories as you thought. Invest in a measuring cup and a food scale, and test your ability to "eyeball" portions from time to time, just to make sure you're staying on target.

Weight Loss Trick #6:

Create a Diversion

Distractions are a good way to keep from overeating. It can take 30-60 minutes to get a "full" sensation, even after a substantial meal. So, after having your "planned" amount of food, get up from the table and get busy! Clean the dishes, do laundry, call a friend, or go for a walk. By the time you're finished, the feeling of fullness should begin to set in, and you will have kept yourself from eating more than you really need.

Weight Loss Trick #7:

Spoil Your Appetite

Fiber can do a lot more than put the bulk back in your bowels. Foods rich in fiber are grrrrrreat for giving you a feeling of fullness. Eating half an apple one hour before dinner will curb your appetite and help you say no to second helpings. Besides fresh fruits, foods high in fiber include beans and fresh crunchy vegetables.

Weight Loss Trick #8:

Pop a Pill???

A number of medications have been shown to be effective for those trying to lose weight and reduce the need for insulin.

ACARBOSE (Precose) is a new medication that slows the digestion of carbohydrates, thus reducing the rise in blood sugar that normally occurs after meals. The combination of weight loss and Acarbose can help eliminate the need for insulin injections. Monitor your blood sugar before and after meals to see if your insulin dose can be reduced.

METFORMIN (Glucophage) is a new medication that enhances the way insulin works. Unlike the older diabetes pills (oral hypoglycemic agents — OHAs), metformin does not make the pancreas produce more insulin. Instead, it helps the insulin you already make work better. Metformin also lowers the amount of sugar released by the liver during the night, resulting in lower blood sugar levels in the morning. In some cases, Metformin can cause mild stomach upset and loss of appetite. But for those trying to lose weight, the loss of appetite can be a welcome side effect.

REDUX (Dexfenfluramine) is an anti-obesity drug that reduces appetite and food cravings. It can be especially helpful when going on a low-calorie diet. There are some potential side effects to Redux, so discuss it with your physician.

TROGLITAZONE. It makes body tissues more sensitive to injected (or your own) insulin that helps you reduce or get rid of insulin or OHA.

Weight Loss Trick #9:

Adjust Your Insulin Program

One or two shots a day may increase your appetite between meals.

The best insulin program for those trying to lose extra weight or maintain the same weight is intermediate-acting insulin (NPH) at bedtime or at supper, and fast-acting insulin (Regular or Humalog) before meals. This type of "multiple injection" program minimizes the total amount of insulin required, and reduces the risk of hypoglycemia. Being on one or two shots of insulin a day means that you are probably taking more insulin than you really need, and will cause you to have a bigger appetite between meals. A multiple injection program allows you to eat less and take less insulin according to the carbohydrate content of your meals. Snacks should not be necessary between meals.

If your present insulin or medication program is causing you to have low blood sugar, it is also forcing you to consume extra calories to treat the low blood sugar. Reducing your dosage to prevent hypoglycemia can help you cut out a hundred calories or more each day.

Weight Loss Trick #10:

Check for Other Medical Conditions

As if having diabetes wasn't enough! Diabetes has been linked with a number of other diseases that can cause weight gain and make it very difficult to lose weight.

Compulsive eating disorders exist in nearly half of all obese people. Binge eating is a disease that may have a physical or psychological basis that can be treated with medication or therapy. Symptoms of binge eating include:

- Eating large quantities of high-calorie foods

- Eating secretively

- Frequent weight fluctuations of more than 10 pounds

- Feeling depressed after eating

- Feeling that you cannot control your eating

Depression is another disorder common among people with diabetes, particularly those who suffer from additional health problems such as diabetic complications. Depression can lead to unhealthy meal patterns and excessive eating. Symptoms include:

- Feeling sad often

- Crying spells

- Tiredness

- Dwelling on negative thoughts

- Dreading the future

- Contemplating suicide

If you are experiencing any of these symptoms, discuss them with your doctor. Once again, there are excellent medications and other forms of therapy for treating depression and reversing these symptoms.

Hypothyroidism, or under-active thyroid, is very common among people who have had diabetes for many years. Thyroid hormone plays a major role in regulating metabolism, so hypothyroidism can make it virtually impossible to lose weight. Symptoms of hypothyroidism include:

- Feeling sluggish

- Decreased appetite

- Slowed reflexes

- Weight gain

- Constipation

- Inability to tolerate cold

Medications for treating hypothyroidism can reverse these symptoms and help restore your metabolism to a normal level.

Key Point:

Many people with diabetes can get off insulin or diabetes pills through healthy living.

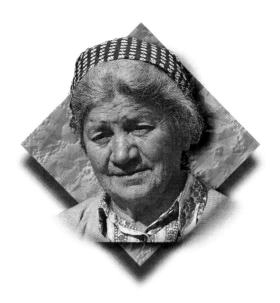

Chapter 17:   Aging With Diabetes

Feeling overlooked and ignored? Seem as if nobody cares about the special problems you face as you age? It is as though somebody is holding a grudge against you just because you were cunning and tough enough to live as long as you have. With most diabetes education programs and materials focusing on juvenile diabetes or obesity-related Type-II diabetes, the special concerns of the elderly are barely touched... until now.

This section is dedicated entirely to nine of the key issues that elderly people with diabetes must face each and every day.

Issue 1: Low blood sugar

Low blood sugar is more common in the elderly than in young people. It is also more dangerous and difficult to treat.

As we age, it is common to miss or skip meals due to lack of appetite, painful arthritis, illness, drowsiness, forgetfulness, or not having enough food in the house. Certain diabetes medications are more difficult to metabolize as we age, and may act longer and stronger than they should. Many people also lose the early warning signs of low blood sugar (shaking, sweating, rapid heartbeat). Instead of recognizing a low blood sugar and treating it with food, it continues to drop until confusion, agitation and poor coordination set in. At this point, it may be difficult to treat low blood sugar on your own.

For all of these reasons, the elderly are at a very high risk of severe low blood sugar. To play it safe, be sure to have your meals on time and in the proper amounts. If necessary, set an alarm clock to remind you of when it is time to eat. Make sure your family, friends and neighbors can recognize the symptoms of low blood sugar (especially abnormal behavior). Teach them how to treat a low blood sugar properly, and always have simple sugar readily available.

Issue 2: Choosing a level of control

Due to the increased risk of severe low blood sugar, special efforts must be made to prevent hypoglycemia in the first place. One way of doing this is by setting appropriate blood sugar "targets."

For example, if you are over age 70, live an active life-style and do not have significant health problems (other than your diabetes), you might aim for blood sugars in the 120-150 range first thing in the morning and before meals. If you are getting readings below 120, you should consider lowering your dose of insulin or diabetes pills (oral hypoglycemic agents - OHAs). If you are disabled and have had major health problems such as a stroke or heart attack, it might be safer to aim for blood sugars in the 150-180 range.

For the elderly, a slightly high reading is much safer than running the risk of low blood sugar.

Issue 3: Multiple medications

Many elderly people take an assortment of medications for a variety of ailments. Even though each medication is important for treating a specific condition, understand that certain combinations can cause problems with diabetes control. Drug interactions are among the most common causes of hospitalization for the elderly.

To minimize the impact of drug interactions, take only those medicines that are absolutely necessary (discuss this with your doctor). Do not start taking an over-the-counter medicine or large dose of vitamins without first discussing it with your doctor. If you take certain medications two or more times a day, ask your doctor or pharmacist if a slow-release (once a day) version is available.

Beware of steroidal medications such as Prednisone. These can cause very high blood sugar and may force you to start taking (or increase your dosage of) insulin. Also, be aware that beta blockers (taken for heart disease or high blood pressure) may slow your recovery from low blood sugar.

Keep a list of all medications you are taking, and update the list every time a drug is added or stopped. If you are seeing more than one physician, make sure every physician knows about all the different drugs you are taking.

Issue 4: Monitoring mishaps

Because the risk of severe hypoglycemia increases with age, the frequency of your monitoring should increase (not decrease) as you age. The more variable your lifestyle, the more often you should check. In other words, if you like to snack, vary meal times, try different foods, dine out, do your own shopping, housework or yardwork, you should be checking your blood sugar several times a day. Frequent blood sugar checks in the middle of the night (3 a.m.) are important for adjusting insulin/medication doses and preventing low blood sugar while you sleep.

By now, you should have discovered that checking blood sugar requires more than just a good finger and a tolerance for pain. It takes the skill to use your meter correctly, including accurate placement of blood on the test strip. With that in mind, look for a meter that is simple to use and has a large, easy-to-read display. Choose a meter with test strips that require only a small amount of blood. Otherwise, it will be difficult to dose the strip properly, and you may wind up with false readings.

If you have difficulty obtaining a good drop of blood, wash your hands with warm water first, and try using a lancing device cap that allows a deeper puncture. Milk your finger for a large drop, and steady your finger with your other hand when placing the drop on the strip.

Issue 5: Difficulties drawing insulin

Apparently, insulin syringes were not designed for people with arthritis or impaired vision. A number of adaptive devices are available to make drawing up insulin a little easier. The Tru-Hand (Whittier Medical - see Appendix B), Count-a-dose (Jordan Medical) and Insul-eze

(Palco Industries) can help magnify and stabilize the syringe and vial so that an accurate dose can be obtained. If you take a small dose of insulin, use syringes with the fewest units possible (25 and 30 unit syringes are available). That way, the number markings and spacings will be as large as possible.

Insulin pens (B-D, Novo-Nordisk) contain prefilled insulin cartridges, so you just dial up your dosage and inject. Needle-free injectors (Health-Mor, MediJect) are another option.

As an alternative, insulin syringes can be pre-filled by a visiting nurse, family member or neighbor so that you just have to reach into the refrigerator and give yourself an injection. Taking things one step further, you could train a family member or hire a visiting nurse to give you the injection at the time you need it. Be careful, though. If you take a combination of fast-acting insulin and Lente or Ultralente insulin, the injection must be given right after the insulin is drawn. Otherwise, the fast acting insulin may lose its potency.

Issue 6: Dietary concerns

They say you can't teach an old dog new tricks. Well, I say the dog wouldn't have lasted this long if it hadn't learned a few tricks along the way.

There is no rule that says you can't enjoy foods that you have always enjoyed. But don't be stubborn and refuse to make any changes to your meal plan. Small, gradual changes can make a big difference in controlling your diabetes, losing weight, and staying healthy.

Remember, food is not your enemy. It is something we all need. You should eat to live, not live to eat. Talk to a dietitian about incorporating some of your favorite foods into a healthy meal plan. And start becoming a label reader. Food companies like to put misleading claims on their packages to get you to buy their products. Read the label for things like carbohydrate (not just sugar) content, grams of fat (not just cholesterol), milligrams of sodium, calories, and portion sizes. That way, you won't be fooled by all the marketing jargon and claims of "sugar free" or "no cholesterol" that are printed on the package.

It is also a good idea to take a complete vitamin/mineral supplement each day. For those who have difficulty chewing, softening your food in a food processor or blender can be helpful. And if you are recovering from an operation or illness, Glucerna is an easily digested food supplement that does not raise blood sugar.

Issue 7: Risk of dizziness and falling

Normally, when a person stands up, their blood pressure holds steady because the blood vessels constrict and the heart speeds up slightly. However, if you have had diabetes for many years or are in poor control, the nerves that normally control blood pressure are slow to respond. The result: you may become dizzy and fall down. Dehydration makes the risk of falling even greater, since blood pressure is more difficult to control when the blood volume is low.

Preventing falls takes more common sense than anything else. Here are a few suggestions:

1. Keep yourself from becoming dehydrated (see the following section).

2. Get up gradually. Before getting out of bed, sit at the edge of the bed and support yourself for a minute or two. This will allow your blood pressure to stabilize before you stand up.

3. Tape down edges of carpets, electrical cords, and any other loose objects that you might trip over.

4. Keep your floors dry and free of objects.

5. Use rubber mats in your bathtub. Install hand bars in the shower and commode areas.

6. Recline after meals or after taking strong heart/blood pressure medication. This can help avoid dizziness due to low blood pressure.

7. Stay home (and out of the sun) for one day when trying a new blood pressure medication or increasing a dosage.

Issue 8: Risk of dehydration

With age, the normal thirst sensation becomes diminished. Your body could be lacking in fluids, and you may not seem the least bit thirsty. People with diabetes are more prone to dehydration because high blood sugar forces us to urinate away fluids rather than retain the fluids we have. If you take diuretics (water pills), you could be at greater risk for dehydration. Caffeine also causes dehydration by forcing you to urinate more.

HYPEROSMOLAR STATE

High blood sugar and dehydration mean that the blood volume will be decreased. This leads to even higher sugar concentrations in the blood. This is a true emergency because it can lead to serious problems with the heart and circulation.

Dehydration can be prevented by:

• Keeping blood sugar levels under 180 as often as possible. Above 180, the kidneys start putting sugar into the urine, which causes extra urination.

- Using diuretics sparingly, and only when absolutely necessary. In most instances, varicose veins and puffy ankles should be treated with compression stockings rather than diuretics.

- Cut down on caffeine consumption.

- Drink plenty of fluids, especially when you are ill or when the weather is hot. If you are cooking in a warm kitchen, drink liquids and try to eat in another area.

- If you need a blood pressure medication, ask for one that is a long-acting, slow-release type.

- Keep the temperature in your home moderate. Jacking up the heat will cause a loss of bodily fluids.

Issue 9: Temperature regulation

Nerve damage is common in elderly people with diabetes. Nerve problems often impair our ability to sense heat, and may make us feel colder than usual. Some people like to turn the thermostat way up. Others like to soak in a hot tub or whirlpool bath. This causes the blood vessels to open up, resulting in a sharp drop in blood pressure. It can also speed the absorption and action of insulin that was previously injected. Elderly people with diabetes should beware of hot environments, because they can cause dangerously low blood pressure, low blood sugar, and dehydration.

Key Point:

Advancing age presents a number of challenges to people with diabetes. Follow your doctor's advice and use common sense to avoid serious accidents and illnesses.

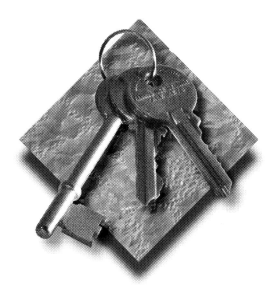

Chapter 18: Emotions and Diabetes

Have you ever been in a very emotional situation? Perhaps someone close to you died or was very sick. Maybe you lost your job and were not sure how you would pay your bills. Possibly you had a fight with your spouse, and he/she walked out. Or maybe you have been mugged or got into a car accident.

When these types of things happen, the last thing you will be concerned about is the state of your diabetes control. After all, crises require your immediate and total attention. If the crisis is short-lived, it may result in only a temporary "blip" in your blood sugar readings. As you will see, this is easily fixed and has minimal long-term effects. But what about emotional issues that don't just pack up and go away?

These can have more far-reaching effects and lead to serious diabetes-related complications in both the short and long-term.

Viper attack vs. Verbal attack

In cave man times, things were pretty simple. There were no in-laws or mortgage payments or busted fax machines to worry about. But there were hungry, cave-man-eating animals with sharp claws and big teeth. The mere sight of these creatures gave the cave man an adrenaline rush so powerful that he could out-run and out-maneuver just about any living creature. The adrenaline rush increases the heart rate and blood pressure, dilates the eyes, tenses the muscles and makes the liver release a jolt of sugar into the bloodstream for quick energy just as we need it.

Unfortunately, our liver can't tell the difference between a "physical" crisis and an "emotional" crisis, so our response to everyday stress is very similar to the response we would get if we were being chased by a bear. You certainly don't need your blood pressure, heart rate and blood sugar to go up every time your transmission slips or you get into an argument. It just happens. Expect to feel tense and have a higher-than-usual blood sugar after an emotionally stressful event.

What you do have control over is your response to stress. Remember, the shorter the period of stress, the less effect it will have on you. In other words, get over it and move on. And if you can predict that a stressful event will take place (i.e. you have a speaking engagement, big test or visit from the in-laws coming up), you can plan your diabetes management accordingly by taking more insulin, eating less, or getting more exercise.

Heck, even a trip to the doctor's office can cause a stress response in many people. You might not think that your friendly, cheerful (and oh so handsome) doctor could cause you to feel stressed, but the mere sight of white labcoats can make some people's blood pressure and blood sugar go up!

Chronic emotional issues

Luckily, most emotionally stressful events are short-lived: Couples kiss and make up. New jobs come along. Fenders get fixed. And time heals most wounds. But emotional stress can become chronic. That is, it lasts a very long time, and shows no signs of letting up. When this happens, emotional stress can literally eat away at your health and happiness.

Depression

One of the most common emotional issues plaguing people with diabetes is depression. Even after diabetes is diagnosed and under relatively good control, reality eventually sets in: The restriction of your favorite foods. Taking shots or pills every day at certain times. Drawing blood from your finger several times a day. The overwhelming nature of having a chronic illness and the unpredictability of blood sugar results often make a person feel that they have lost control of some important parts of their life. You may have a constant fear of the long-term complications, or may already have complications. Research has shown that the more complications a person has, the greater their chances of also being depressed.

Depression doesn't just mean "having the blues." We all get the blues from time to time, but the symptoms go away. Depression lingers like smog over a big city. It is usually due to a chemical imbalance in the brain, similar to the way a lack of insulin causes diabetes. It is not caused by anything you did or did not do; it is a medical condition that, like diabetes, requires treatment.

Depression can affect you in many ways. Some people with depression cry a lot; others don't cry at all. It can cause you to be irritable, tired all the time or pessimistic. It can change your appetite so that you binge or hardly eat at all. Any setback or stressful situation could make you withdraw or put you in a horrible mood. Other symptoms include difficulty sleeping, headaches and weakness.

Depression can wreak havoc on your health, happiness, sense of well-being, relationships and career. It can also screw up your blood sugar control by affecting your eating habits, keeping you from exercising, and generally making you less interested in taking good care of yourself. High blood sugars will make you feel even worse, which could make the depression more severe.

IF YOU THINK YOU MIGHT BE DEPRESSED, SEE A HEALTH PROFESSIONAL AND GET IT TREATED. Depression is a treatable condition, but until you get it treated, very little can be done to improve your state of mind or your diabetes control. Depression is like a wall that surrounds you; you have to break through the wall before you can be treated for anything else.

Treatment for depression is better than ever before. Nobody wants to take more pills than they have to, but today's anti-depression drugs (including Zoloft, Prozac and Paxil) are fast, effective, and relatively free of side effects. The difference in people who start using these medications is unbelievable.

Whether or not you are diagnosed with depression, try to remember that there are some things about diabetes we can control, and some things we can't. If you dwell on the things you can't control, it will keep you from doing what you need to do today. A baseball player who is too busy kicking himself for striking out his last time up is not likely to get a hit in his next at bat. Deep in your heart, you must believe that control of diabetes matters, and that there are many things you can do to improve your control and ultimately prevent complications.

Insomnia

Insomnia simply means trouble falling asleep. It could be due to stress in your daily life that won't let you unwind or relax. It could also be caused by caffeine intake.

Staying awake, in and of itself, is not a problem for people with diabetes. The problem is what we do when we are awake at night. Many people will read or watch TV... and munch, and munch, and munch. It is easy to eat way too much when you are not paying attention to what you are doing, and this often happens late at night. The result is high blood sugar which might wake you up later to run to the bathroom. And if you stay up late and munch often enough, you might start to put on weight.

There are a number of methods for overcoming insomnia. Progressive relaxation (deep breathing, tightening and then relaxing each muscle individually) at bedtime can help you to escape the stresses of the day and put you in the right frame of body and mind for going to sleep. Cutting down on caffeine (or only having caffeine in the morning) may also help. Evening exercise can also make it more difficult to fall asleep. Try exercising in the morning instead.

Chronic stress

We all know the type. He (or she) is a perfectionist, works non-stop, and is constantly tired and frustrated about something. Chronic (long-term) stress is a bad dream that doesn't go away. Worse than the way it can make you feel, chronic stress can cause damage all over your body - ulcers in the stomach, a weakened immune system, headaches, chest pain, and our old friend high blood sugar.

Remember, stress signals the liver to release sugar into the bloodstream. Chronic stress means that your liver is going to be raising your blood sugar often and in unpredictable amounts. Talk about a challenge to your diabetes control!

Chronic stress is usually caused by a negative interpretation of the situation we are in. For example, let's look at two salespeople: Bob and Rick. Both work for the same organization, doing the same work in the same office for the same pay at the same time. Bob is constantly "stressed out" by the workload, frustrated with his co-workers, and is worried about his future. Rick seems to enjoy his work. He does what he can and hopes for the best results. He jokes about the impossible workload, and generally takes things in stride. Same situations, two different interpretations.

If the stresses of daily living have you feeling wiped out, talk it over with a Psychologist or Psychiatrist. They can't change your situation, but they may be able to help you see it in a different light.

Anxiety

"Anxiety" is another word for fear. Fear elicits a stress response similar to most stress responses, including a rapid heartbeat and sudden release of sugar into the bloodstream. Some people experience severe responses to anxiety; these are called "panic attacks."

Fear is really a good thing - it keeps us from doing stupid things (like jumping off cliffs) and lets us respond quickly to dangerous situations. However, anxiety over common, everyday events or situations is similar to chronic stress - it can cause frequent and unpredictable rises in blood sugar. And for people with heart disease or other complications of diabetes, the body's extreme response to fear can lead to a worsening of the complication.

Anxiety is treatable through psychotherapy, medication (tranquilizers), or a combination of the two. If you feel that anxiety may present a challenge to your diabetes control, be sure to discuss it with your doctor.

Compulsive eating

Unlike "overeating," which is a conscious act of eating more than you really should, "compulsive eating" is caused by subconscious drives that are beyond your control. Often, compulsive eating is due to an unresolved psychological conflict (such as difficulty living with or accepting diabetes or its complications) or the need to release anger or aggression. Compulsive eating is destructive and should be treated as soon as possible.

If you find yourself eating often (even when you are not hungry), eating in response to stress, or simply feel that you have lost your ability to say "no" to food, talk to your doctor or a skilled therapist.

Key point:

Diabetes is a physically and emotionally demanding disease that requires a focused effort to control. If you suspect that you have an emotional problem that might get in the way of your diabetes management, don't hesitate to have it evaluated and treated.

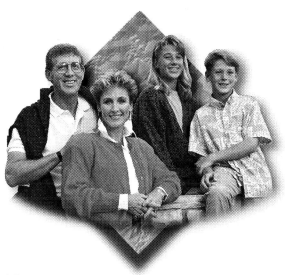

Chapter 19:
Family, Friends and Co-Workers (Oh, My!)

Sometimes, we all have thoughts of getting away from people, going to live alone on a desert island where nobody can nag us or give us a hard time. Before you go out to buy a boat, remember this: loneliness is a terrible thing. In many cases, isolation is used as a form of punishment. Why do you think your parents made you go to your room when you behaved badly? It was to leave you alone with your guilty conscience. Face it. People need people. In the words of singer/songwriter Chrissie Hynde:

"The reason we're here as man and woman, is to love eachother.

Help each other. Stand by each other."

To be human is to relate to other people. We all know how complex and challenging human relations can be. Adding diabetes to the mix is like throwing sparks near a tank of gasoline. Sooner or later, something is bound to explode.

The explosion may take place at home because your spouse is trying to control every morsel of food you put in your mouth. It might happen with friends who treat you like an invalid just because you take shots. Or it could happen at work because the workload is forcing you to be late for lunch and miss your evening workouts. Learning to deal effectively with the people around you will help to not only put out the explosions, but prevent them from ever getting started.

Assigning responsibility

Take a moment to walk over to the mirror. Say to yourself three times, "I am responsible for my diabetes care." Good. Now that we have that out of the way, we can get down to business.

Too many people like to pin responsibility for their health concerns on their doctors, spouses, family members, or even their insurance companies. YOU are ultimately responsible for taking care of yourself. The sooner you come to accept that, the sooner you can take control of your health and your life.

Of course, there are special exceptions. Very young children must rely on their parents to make daily decisions about food, insulin doses, activity and so on. Those who have mental impairments may require the guidance and assistance of a skilled nurse or family member. *Physical* impairment does not excuse you from taking responsibility for your diabetes. You may need to obtain special equipment or outside assistance for performing routine tasks, but decision making and accountability fall squarely on your shoulders.

What your spouse/partner should know

Just because you are responsible for your diabetes care doesn't mean that you go about it alone. Think of yourself as the coach of a football team. You still need players to go out and help you win the big game.

Your spouse (husband, wife, roommate, life-partner) is kind of like your quarterback. You might be making the calls and directing the flow of the game, but the quarterback is very important for helping carry out your game plan. When your diabetes seems to get overwhelming, your spouse should be able to step in and help you do the job.

Don't forget, diabetes requires a lot of changes for the entire family. It took you some time to adjust to all these changes, so give your spouse the same slack. Talk to your spouse about your diabetes - how you feel about it, and what you need to do to control it. Distancing your diabetes from your spouse will only make the adjustment more difficult for both of you.

Over time, there are many things your spouse should learn about and be able to do. Many of these can be learned from your doctor, diabetes educator, classes at a local hospital, or from reading books and magazines about diabetes.

1. How to check your blood sugar with a monitor. You may need help checking your blood sugar while you are very sick, sleeping or have lost consciousness (possibly due to low blood sugar).

2. The types and quantity of medications and supplies you use. Your spouse may need to order supplies for you. They can also keep an eye out to make sure you don't run out of an important item such as insulin or test strips.

3. How and when to give a glucagon injection. This could save your life in the event of severe hypoglycemia. See chapter 14 for details.

4. <u>Nutritional content of foods prepared at home</u>. Your spouse should be aware of the role carbohydrates, fat, calories and salt play in your diabetes management, and should know how to prepare meals that fit within your meal plan. Whoever prepares the meals at home should try to prepare them in a healthy manner, using as little fat as possible. A willingness to cut down on meat consumption can be a definite plus.

5. <u>Important names and phone numbers</u>. In an emergency, your spouse should be able to contact your physician, pharmacy, diabetes educator or local hospital at a moment's notice.

6. <u>Symptoms and treatment for low blood sugar</u>. Low blood sugar is a fact of life for most people with diabetes. Even the most well-controlled person will occasionally experience hypoglycemia. Some people, especially those who have had diabetes for many years or who control their blood sugars very intensively, do not get the usual symptoms of low blood sugar (shaking, sweating, rapid heartbeat), and may not realize that their blood sugar is low until confusion sets in. The spouse and rest of the family need to know:

   A. When to suspect low blood sugar (after exercise, and with a delayed meal),

   B. What the symptoms are (symptoms can range from obvious physical signs such as trembling, sweating or cold/pale skin to subtle behaviors such as slurred speech, irritability, a confused look, poor coordination (tripping, dropping things), or simply acting unusual), and

   C. How to treat it (1/2 cup of juice or regular soda, 3-4 glucose tablets, or whatever you have designated as your "official food of hypoglycemic reactions"), and where it can be found.

Low blood sugar should be explained to all members of the family in a serious tone. The way a person looks or acts when their blood sugar is low is deadly serious; it is not funny. If not treated properly, it can lead to coma or death. Your spouse should be prepared to do any driving necessary until your blood sugar returns to normal after an episode of low blood sugar.

7. How to recognize a heart attack. Because people with diabetes are at a very high risk for heart disease and may not feel any pain if a heart attack occurs, the spouse should know how to recognize symptoms of a heart attack or stroke. These include chest pain/pressure, left shoulder pain, arm pain, sweating, shortness of breath, loss of balance, or other unusual behaviors. If you have a history of heart disease, your spouse should assist you with blood pressure monitoring and should learn how to do CPR (cardiopulmonary resuscitation).

8. How to inject insulin. Your spouse should know how to give injections in hard-to-reach places such as the buttocks or back of the arms. This will give you more sites to choose from, and can reduce your risk of lipodystrophy.

LIPODYSTROPHY

When injections are given repeatedly in the same part of the body, the fat tissue below the skin can become damaged. The area may become hard, swollen, bumpy, or indented. Insulin will not absorb well from this site, and may result in high blood sugar levels.

---

9. Encourage you to exercise. Exercise is important for weight loss as well as daily blood sugar control. Your spouse can help by giving you the time to exercise, getting you the right workout clothes or equipment, or even joining you in your workouts. Exercising with someone makes it more fun!

10. <u>Assist with foot inspections</u>. A daily foot exam is critical for catching minor injuries before they become serious. If you have impaired vision or have difficulty examining the tops and bottoms of your feet, have your spouse check them for cuts, abrasions, calluses, blisters, and foreign objects.

What your spouse/partner should <u>not</u> do

<u>Assume control</u>. It is completely understandable that your spouse will want to do everything possible to help you control your diabetes. But remember, responsibility for your diabetes care is yours. Others can support and encourage, but letting someone else try to control your diabetes for you is a major conflict waiting to happen. Changes are in order if your spouse starts to do any of the following:

<u>Encourage overeating when blood sugar is low</u>. A period of hypoglycemia is one of those times when cooler heads must prevail. The temptation is always there to keep feeding a person with low blood sugar until the symptoms go away, but this will not speed recovery from a low blood sugar and will only cause problems later on. Educate your spouse on proper treatment of low blood sugar, and emphasize the specific types and amounts of foods required to treat it.

<u>Lock you into the same foods day after day</u>. Variety truly is the spice of life. The meal plan for most people with diabetes simply involves limiting fat intake and matching carbohydrate amounts to insulin levels. Increasing fiber intake and lowering salt intake are also key components in many cases. This is much healthier than the usual American diet, and it still allows a great deal of freedom and flexibility.

<u>Expect perfection</u>. None of us IS perfect. Explain to your spouse that diabetes is not an exact science, and things may not turn out right all

the time. As long as you are truly giving it your best, that is all that anyone, including your spouse, can expect.

Obsess over numbers. Numbers can exert powerful control over the emotional lives of you and your spouse. Beautiful mornings and special moments can be ruined in the time it takes to monitor your blood sugar. Numbers should be viewed as a means for improving control rather than the "goal". Your blood sugar results can be used as a tremendous learning tool for making adjustments and learning "what works, and what doesn't". Let your numbers work for you, not own you.

Tradition vs. Prescription

There are times when recommendations given by your doctor or diabetes educators conflict with traditions held by you and your family. The diet, in particular, plays a key role in many families. Changing the diet should be a family decision, because the whole family needs to get involved. It is very difficult (and unfair) to ask a person with diabetes to follow a separate diet from the rest of the family. As mentioned earlier, the diet that is recommended for someone with diabetes is much better than the typical American diet. It would benefit the entire family to start eating healthier.

It is best to modify the existing diet than change it completely. For example, the Hispanic diet usually has plenty of protein, carbohydrate and fiber (due to beans). This diet can be improved simply by having modest portion sizes and broiling rather than frying. The Oriental diet typically contains a great deal of rice and foods high in salt. Once again, portion sizes need to be checked since rice contains a great deal of carbohydrate, and salt intake (from MSG and other sources) needs to be reduced.

Obesity creates another dilemma. In some cultures, heaviness is a sign of success, power, dignity and style. Type-II diabetes runs very high in Hispanic-American, African-American, and Native-American cultures. High blood pressure and complications such as kidney disease are also very common in these populations. We know for a fact that weight loss and exercise can prevent and control Type-II diabetes. It is not necessary to give up traditional values, but a little bit of compromise could save your life.

In certain cultures, tradition calls for fasting. Fasting is possible for those who use an insulin pump, but it can be very dangerous for those who take insulin injections or diabetes pills (oral hypoglycemic agents). Most religions recognize the medical need for people with diabetes to eat and approve of it, even on Holy days.

In many families, the "head of the household" is a proud and honorary position. Some people think that having diabetes or needing help to control it are signs of weakness. On the contrary, it is a sign of STRENGTH! The very fact that you can lead your family despite having a challenging chronic illness shows how resilient and resourceful you are. And the ability to organize the people around you to assist with various parts of your diabetes management is a true sign of leadership.

Families that are used to chowing down the moment they reach the table may need to wait a few minutes to allow for blood sugar checks, insulin injections, and so on. When insulin is to be given prior to a meal, the person preparing the meal should notify the person with diabetes well ahead of time about the meal contents (so carbohydrates can be estimated) and the approximate time the meal will be ready (so insulin injections can be timed appropriately).

The power of communication

Friends and family members should be told openly that you did not do anything bad to get diabetes; it just happened. There is no shame in having diabetes, just as there is no shame in wearing eyeglasses to correct faulty vision. Silence on your part is the one thing that will make people suspicious and treat you "differently". Talking about your diabetes and educating those around you will make living with diabetes safer and more pleasant. It will also aid in your ongoing acceptance of the disease.

The "diabetic" label

Some of us like to play basketball from time to time. But that doesn't mean that we go around introducing ourselves as a basketball players (unless, of course, your name happens to be Michael Jordan).

Do not identify yourself, or allow yourself to be identified, as a "diabetic". You are a complex person with many interests and characteristics, only one of which is diabetes. Labels like "diabetic" often dictate how we act, think and feel. They reduce you to a set of behaviors or beliefs held by the people around you. By rejecting the "diabetic" label, you will get others to treat you as an individual.

Rights & responsibilities in the workplace

In the workplace, you have certain rights that are guaranteed by the Constitution as well as fair trade practices. Employers cannot discriminate against you because you have diabetes. This applies to hiring, promotion, pay, training, and firing. There are a few special exceptions, however: For safety reasons, <u>a person with diabetes who takes</u>

insulin cannot be an air traffic controller or fly a plane; and in some states, you may not be able to obtain a license to be a truck driver or operate any commercial vehicle.

The Americans with Disabilities Act states that reasonable accommodations must be made for people with disabilities if those accommodations would allow you to perform essential functions of the job. If you need to eat, check your blood, or take an injection at certain times, your employer must allow you to do so. You should expect to be treated with dignity and fairness. If you feel that you have been treated unfairly due to your diabetes, you should contact your local chapter of the American Civil Liberties Union.

With your rights come some responsibility on your part. It is strongly recommended that you do the following:

1. Let your employer know that you have diabetes and what you need to do to keep it well-controlled.

2. Educate your supervisor and co-workers about the symptoms and treatment of low blood sugar.

3. Keep treatment for low blood sugar (glucose tablets, etc.) in a readily-accessible place. Let a co-worker know where it is.

4. Avoid using diabetes as an excuse for not performing your job properly.

5. Do not leave hazardous materials (syringes, lancets, medications) in garbage cans or accessible places. Keep them locked up and dispose of them in a proper container.

6. Work smart. Plan your schedule so you can take your insulin/medications, meals, and blood sugar tests at the proper times. Delays can lead to hypoglycemia.

7. Keep your blood sugar under the best control possible. High blood sugar levels can make you drowsy and may impair your

ability to think clearly. Your employer deserves you at your absolute best!

Tips for handling conflicts

Inevitably, conflicts will arise from time to time. The way you handle conflicts can make the difference between mountains and molehills.

First, recognize that conflict is the result of an underlying problem. Identify the problem and what you want to change. Negotiate changes (each side may have to give a little bit), and reward both sides when progress is made. This way, you turn a potential negative into a positive.

Things that happened in the past are often the source of conflict. It is important to allow the past to stay where it is - in the past. We are not condemned to repeat what has happened in the past. You have free will and the benefit of experience. Use the past to live better now and have hope for tomorrow.

Key point:

Diabetes affects more than just the person who has it. You are responsible for your diabetes care, but look to your spouse, family, friends and co-workers for support.

Chapter 20:   Health Insurance

Insurance. One word that makes teeth grind. Blood boil. Veins pop out in heads. And with good reason: The current state of health insurance can be very frustrating and unfair to people with diabetes. Considering how expensive it can be to manage your diabetes, you owe it to yourself to find out all you can about how your health insurance operates. That way, you may be able to get a much larger chunk of your diabetes care costs covered.

The cost of diabetes care

Personal health and well-being aside, the financial cost of diabetes is staggering. More than 50 billion dollars is spent each year treating diabetes and its complications. Another 50 billion dollars is lost through diabetes-related illness, disability and death. Overall, more than 10% of all health costs in the U.S. are related to diabetes. On average, a person with diabetes now costs his or her insurance company more than $9000 a year, most of it due to treating long-term complications. If you had to pay for all of your diabetes care costs out of pocket, you would probably wind up broke. That is why we need health insurance.

The current state of health insurance

The main purpose of health insurance is to spread risk around so that nobody carries a heavy burden all alone. If one person gets seriously ill, they would not be able to afford to pay for their care. However, by having health insurance, the cost is absorbed by many policyholders who each pay for coverage. In the past, this system worked pretty well. Health professionals (doctors, hospitals, etc.) provided the service, and insurance companies dealt out the dollars and cents.

Today, all of that has changed. In our current "managed care" system, insurance companies still control the dollars and cents, but many are also dictating where you must go for health care and what kind of care you can receive. Actually, you can still go anywhere you want and get whatever you want, but you may have to pay for it out of your own pocket. And with health care costs as high as they are, this is not an option for most people.

By controlling access to health care, insurance companies feel that they can still provide adequate care without the waste and abuse that tends to drive health care costs up.

HMOs, or Health Maintenance Organizations, are networks of health providers (physicians, podiatrists, hospitals, pharmacies, laboratories, etc.). You are required to use health providers in the network in order to have the products and services paid for by the company. Often, a PCP (Primary Care Physician) directs your overall care. The PCP determines if and when you need to see a specialist, and what special products or services may be necessary for your health.

PPOs, or Preferred Provider Organizations, are similar to HMOs, except that they usually cover a portion of the products and services you receive from out-of-network providers. You are not usually required to get the permission of a PCP before seeing a specialist with a PPO.

Before, the incentive in the health care industry was to make as much money as possible from taking care of sick people. More doctors visits, more tests, and more hospitalizations meant that the health care providers made more money. Now, the incentive is on getting people well and keeping them well for as little money as possible. The less the managed care organization has to spend taking care of you, the more of your premium (the amount you or your employer spends for your coverage) it can keep for itself.

That, too, has its problems. Some managed care organizations make it difficult for you to get reimbursement or access to diabetes supplies, health education, and screenings to prevent major complications. This is where your savvy and expertise in dealing with insurance companies can help a great deal.

Your primary needs: how to choose the best insurance plan

In almost all cases, you have a choice of insurance plans with which you can subscribe. First of all, you should make every effort to join as part of a group plan through your employer, a local chamber of commerce, or an association. As a person with diabetes, it will be very difficult for you to obtain a good health insurance policy on your own. Any policy you get will probably exclude coverage for the treatment of diabetes, limit your benefits, or charge you extremely high premiums. When you join a group plan, an HMO cannot refuse coverage to people with pre-existing conditions.

In many states, Blue Cross/Blue Shield and some HMOs offer "open enrollment" periods for health insurance. You do not have to be part of a group to sign up during open enrollment. But be aware that policies offered during open enrollment usually do not cover as much as policies obtained through a group.

If you are having difficulties with your insurance company or want to find out about state-subsidized health insurance plans for children, insurance risk-pools or other opportunities for obtaining health insurance, contact your State Insurance Commissioner's Office.

Usually, a group such as an employer will offer a few different insurance options. The best plan is the one that meets most of your primary needs as a person with diabetes. These will probably include:

- A doctor with whom you are comfortable. If you already see a certain doctor for your diabetes care, it is best to join the plan that the doctor is part of.

- Coverage for diabetes education. This can include group education classes or one-on-one visits with dietitians and Certified Diabetes Educators.

- Coverage for diabetes supplies, especially "disposable" items like blood sugar test strips and insulin syringes.

- A prescription plan that will cover your diabetes medications such as insulin and diabetes pills.

- Easy access to specialists, including renal specialists (for treating kidney disease), Ophthalmologists (for diagnosing and treating eye problems), Podiatrists (for maintaining foot care), Neurologists (for treating nerve problems), and cardiac specialists in the event of heart problems.

- Always choose the option that offers the lowest deductibles and smallest co-payments. Taking care of diabetes can get expensive, so look for a policy that covers as much as possible.

What is *usually* covered

Gone are the days of blanket, across-the-board coverage for everything you need to manage and treat your diabetes. In order to make a profit, managed care organizations try to keep you healthy and functional for as little cost as possible.

Different insurance policies provide different levels of care. Medicare, for example, will reimburse you 80% of the cost of the following, once your deductible has been met:

- A blood glucose meter
- Blood sugar test strips
- A lancet device
- Lancets
- Therapeutic shoes
- Laser surgery for retinopathy
- Dialysis
- Lab tests (100% covered)
- Diabetes education (in approved programs)

To qualify for Medicare reimbursement of these items/services, you must be over 65 (or have advanced kidney disease), be taking insulin, and have a letter of medical necessity from your doctor. Medicare does not cover insulin, syringes, insulin pumps, routine eye exams and foot care, or blood sugar testing supplies for those who do not take insulin.

For obtaining your diabetes supplies, Medicare has its own list of "participating" pharmacies and supply houses. Getting your supplies through these businesses can save you money because the prices they charge must be approved by Medicare. Under federal law, the pharmacy or supply company is required to submit your claim forms to Medicare for you. For more information on what Medicare does and does not pay for, you can obtain "The Medicare Handbook" for $3 from the Superintendent of Documents in Washington, DC (see Appendix B).

Among private insurance companies, coverage for diabetes supplies and services varies a great deal. Make a list of all the supplies and services you think you might need to keep your diabetes well-controlled, and either read your policy carefully or call the insurance company's customer service department to find out the specific level of coverage for each item on your list.

How to save money on your diabetes care

Let's say you are at the mall, shopping for a sweater. Two stores have virtually identical sweaters - one store sells it for $49, the other for $39. So, you go back to the first store and tell the manager that you would like to buy the sweater there, but she will have to beat the second store's price. The manager is so eager to keep your business that you wind up taking the sweater home for a mere 30 bucks. Consider the $19 savings a fair return for being a smart shopper.

When it comes to buying diabetes supplies and services, you also have to be a smart shopper. Never forget that you are the customer, and you deserve to be treated fairly. Sometimes, you might have to be persistent and do some negotiating to get what you want, but the rewards make it worth the effort.

Here are a few ways you can cut your out-of-pocket costs for diabetes products and professional services:

1. Shop around for over-the-counter items like meters and test strips. Some mail-order pharmacies (listed in the back of popular diabetes magazines) offer products at substantial discounts over retail.

2. Buying in bulk can save you money. Instead of purchasing 25 test strips at a time, buy boxes of 100 or more.

3. Submit claim forms for all the diabetes-related products and professional health services you receive. The worst that can happen is that your claim is rejected. At best, you will receive a handsome check in the mail.

4. If a claim is rejected, have your doctor write a strong letter of medical necessity for every diabetes product and service you require. Send this, along with a copy of the original prescription and your claim form, back to your insurance company.

5. To make your claim even stronger, include a letter from the your doctor or diabetes educator specifying how much better you are doing since the service was provided.

6. Use the right language in claim forms and letters/prescriptions. "Education" and "counseling" are typically frowned upon by insurance companies. Terms like "Therapy" and "Diabetes Management" are much more likely to receive approval.

7. Persistence counts! Even if claims have not been approved in the past, keep submitting them in the future. Policies may have changed, or you might just get lucky.

A final word...

Remember in the last chapter when we talked about responsibility? Specifically, about not placing responsibility for your diabetes care on anyone but yourself? That means you can't rely on your insurance company to pay for everything you need to take care of yourself. The main benefit of insurance is the same as it was years ago: It will help take care of you in case of a very costly problem. When it comes to the day-to-day stuff, you may have to assume some of the financial responsibility on your own. That includes diabetes education, monitoring supplies, exercise equipment, healthy food, dietary counseling, quality footwear and foot care, and anything else that can improve your diabetes control.

Considering that you only have one body and one life, think of it as an investment for a longer and better future.

Key point:

Be a smart shopper when dealing with insurance companies and coverage of diabetes services and supplies.

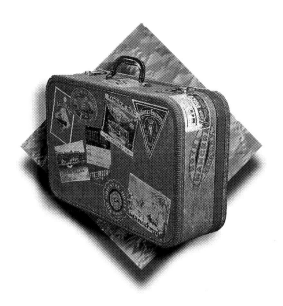

Chapter 21: Travel: Diabetes On The Go

Things sure ain't what they used to be, partner. Back in the "good ol' days", everyone y'all knew and everything y'all needed - buddies, kin, customers, the sheriff, Doc Holiday, the general store — were all within walking distance of the old homestead. "Travel" meant a stagecoach ride to the next town to buy wood or goats or something else useful.

Today, extended travel is a part of everyday life. Friends, family, businesses and vacation spots are spread so far apart that many people find themselves "on the road" almost as often as they are at home. Having diabetes should not stand in the way of your travels, but it does present some special situations and challenges to your diabetes care. Nobody wants to wind up in an emergency room when they travel, so follow the old Boy Scout motto: **BE PREPARED!**

WHAT TO PREPARE FOR

Travel can present some special challenges for people with diabetes. The key is to prepare for these challenges before they occur.

Sunburn is common whenever people travel, especially if you plan to be outdoors a lot. Due to neuropathy, you may not feel sunburn coming on until it is quite severe. Use sunscreen, sunglasses and a hat when you plan to be outdoors.

Foot injuries are another common occurrence during travel, particularly if you plan to do a lot of walking. A trip is no time to start wearing a new pair of shoes. Wear comfortable, broken-in walking shoes and thick cotton socks when walking. Be careful not to walk barefooted on hot sand and pavement. As always, check your feet daily for redness, blisters, cuts and scrapes.

Due to changes in meals, activity and schedules, blood sugars may change quite a bit when you travel. You should monitor a little bit more than usual to see if you need to make any adjustments. Be careful with your meter because not every machine gives accurate readings at high altitudes. Some meters are also affected by very high or low temperatures. Check your owner's manual to see if your meter may be affected when you travel.

When you are away from home, meals may be delayed or unavailable. Physical activity is often increased due to all the walking you must do. These factors can lead to low blood sugar. The principle of eating extra food when you are active becomes more important than ever.

On days when you are traveling through time zones, it is best to stop using intermediate and long-acting insulins (NPH, Lente, Ultralente) and switch to only rapid-acting insulins (regular or Humalog). Check your blood sugar every four hours while in transit, and give yourself rapid-acting insulin according to how much food you plan to eat and how high your blood sugar is. Your doctor can help you figure the appropriate doses for your trip.

Keep your watch set at its usual time while you are in transit. Once you have arrived at your destination and are ready for bed, you can adjust your watch to the local time and return to your usual insulin program. On the return trip, go once again to the rapid-insulin-only schedule, and don't go back to your usual insulin program or change your watch until you arrive home and are ready for bed.

Remember, travel to the North or South does not affect time zones. Traveling East will shorten the day, so you will probably need less insulin than usual. Traveling West will lengthen the day, so you will probably need more insulin than usual. If you are only crossing one or two time zones (gaining/losing one or two hours), you probably won't need to make any major adjustments. Longer travel, especially travel overseas, will require more changes to your usual routine.

When traveling by car, it is common for blood sugar levels to run higher than usual. You may need to cut back on your carbohydrates or increase your insulin on the day of a trip. It is also a good idea to stop at least every two hours and take a brisk walk. This will help improve your circulation and let your insulin do a better job of lowering your blood sugar.

Of course, rest stops are ideal times to check your blood sugar. Keep non-perishable food in your glove compartment (glucose tablets, peanut butter crackers, juice in cans or boxes) in case of an emergency. It is never safe to operate a car when your blood sugar is low; your reaction times and depth perception will be impaired. If you become hypoglycemic, pull off the road and treat the low blood sugar with simple carbohydrate and a protein snack, such as Life Savers and peanut butter crackers. Although your blood sugar may rise in 15 minutes, it will take your brain longer to get back to normal, so give yourself a good 30-60 minutes before driving again.

If possible, keep a cellular phone in the car, along with phone numbers for your doctor and roadside assistance. In an emergency, a cellular phone could save your life.

When traveling by plane, Murphy's law applies: Whatever can go wrong, will (probably) go wrong.

What can go wrong when you fly? Plenty. Luggage can be lost or misplaced, so bring a complete set of all your diabetes supplies and medications in your carry-on baggage. Flights are often delayed, so bring your own food or prepare to have a snack at the airport.

On-flight meals can also present a problem. Airline food is notoriously dry and unhealthy, so order a special "diabetic meal" ahead of time. Of course, there is no such thing as a "diabetic meal." But the airlines don't know that. They often prepare meals that are heartier and healthier for people with medical conditions, so go for it. Also, don't count on your food arriving at your seat at any particular time. Wait until the food is placed in front of you before taking your insulin. Of course this is not ideal, but better to have your blood sugar run a little high after the meal than to risk hypoglycemia while waiting for a slow steward to make his way down the aisle.

Due to the dryness onboard most planes, drink as much as you can get your hands on (sugar-free if possible). Stay away from caffeinated drinks since they can cause extra urination, and try not to drink alcohol since it may lead to low blood sugar later in the night (see Chapter 22).

If your flight lasts for several hours, get up and walk around as often as you can. This will help improve your circulation and get your insulin to work a little better.

If you need to take an insulin injection on a plane, only inject half as much air as usual into the vial. Cabin pressure is lower than the air pressure on the ground, so you won't need to build up as much pressure inside the bottle.

When going on a cruise, ask for information on the ports of call, climates, menus, activities, and medical care available on-board. Most cruise ships have a doctor on board. Give a summary of your medical history to the doctor at the beginning of the cruise so that he/she will be prepared in case you have any problem. Because you are likely to eat more than usual on a cruise, make sure you practice counting carbohydrates and using a sliding scale for your insulin doses prior to the trip.

WHAT TO BRING

- Medical ID: When you travel, always wear medical identification, stating that you have diabetes and what you take to treat it. A wallet card and Medic Alert bracelet or necklace (Medic Alert Foundation, see Appendix B) can save your life in case you lose consciousness or are in an accident.

- Prescriptions from your doctor for all of your medications and diabetes-related supplies.

- A letter from your doctor indicating that you have diabetes and must take insulin (or medication) and check your blood sugar levels. The letter should include a list of your medications, allergies, past and present illnesses, and blood type.

- Sinus medicine: Stuffy sinuses can be unbearably painful when flying in a plane, especially if the cabin pressure is not well maintained. If you have a history of sinus problems, bring a sinus medication with you.

- Medicine for treating diarrhea and upset stomach, such as Imodium and Pepto Bismol. Also, if you are prone to motion sickness, bring an effective medication such as Meclizine.

- An extra pair of sunglasses or contact lenses: It is easy to lose or damage a pair when you travel.

- Your blood glucose meter with extra batteries, and enough lancets and test strips to last twice as long as your trip is expected to take.

- Ketone-testing strips for use if you become ill.

- Twice as many bottles of insulin and syringes (or diabetes pills) as you expect to need.

- Glucagon in case you have severe low blood sugar and lose consciousness. Make sure someone you are traveling with knows how and when to use glucagon.

- Your doctor's phone number: In non-emergency situations, your physician back home is your best source of advice.

- A few Band-Aids as well as over-the-counter antibiotic ointment for minor cuts.

- Non-perishable food, such as Life Savers, glucose tablets, or cans of juice.

If you usually use an insulin pump or jet injector, bring syringes with you just in case you have a mechanical problem. If you use a jet injector, bring extra vial adapters. If you use an insulin pump, bring extra batteries and twice as many syringes/infusion sets as you expect to use. A waterproof case for your pump may be necessary if you plan to be in or around water.

To carry your supplies, it is a good idea to invest in a carrying case specially designed for people with diabetes, such as the DiaPak (Atwater Carey) or MedPort (MedPort, Inc.) carrying cases - see Appendix B. Some cases include a gel freezer pack that keeps your insulin and medications cool while you travel. Remember, it is OK to keep your insulin at room temperature, but you should not expose your insulin to freezing temperatures or temperatures over 86 degrees Fahrenheit. <u>Never</u> leave your insulin in the car. Medicool's Insulin Protector and Palco Labs' InsulTote (see Appendix B) are excellent insulated carrying cases for times when you are outdoors hiking, in the tropics, on the beach, or anyplace where your insulin may be exposed to high temperatures.

INTERNATIONAL TRAVEL

When traveling in another country, you are not going to find the same quality medical care and clean conditions you have come to expect at home. Be prepared for just about anything. There are 84 countries that have diabetes associations that can help you plan your travel. For a copy of the list, or to subscribe to <u>The Diabetic Traveler</u> (a quarterly newsletter designed to help people with diabetes plan safe and secure travel), contact The Diabetic Traveler (see Appendix B).

Be aware that insulin outside the U.S. could have a different concentration than the U-100 insulin you are used to using. It is common to find U-40 insulin, which means that the insulin is only 40% as potent as U-100 insulin. If you run out of your insulin and are forced to use U-40 insulin, multiply your usual dose by 2 1/2. In other words, if you usually take 10 units of NPH insulin (U-100), you will need 25 units of NPH insulin that is U-40 to get the same effect.

If you are in a non-English speaking country, carry a card that has "I have diabetes" translated into the local language. It is also a good idea to write down a few phrases in the native language in case you need to ask for orange juice, seek medical care, or explain that you have low blood sugar.

Always be suspicious of water and raw foods in foreign countries. Even if you are told that the food and water are perfectly safe, enough people have become sick to say otherwise. Here are a few tips:

- Do not eat anything bought from street vendors.

- Stay away from milk and dairy products.

- Drink carbonated water rather than tap water or mineral water. The carbonation should get rid of any bacteria that may have been in the water.

- Avoid ice cubes made from the local water. If you want to cool down a drink, put the ice cubes in a plastic bag and place the bag in your drink.

- Peel your own fruits and melons. Do non trust pre-peeled fruits.

- Look for cooked rather than raw vegetables.

Remember, dinner in foreign countries is often served later than in the U.S., and you may also have difficulty getting diet soft drinks.

GOD FORBID...

If you find yourself in the middle of nowhere and do not have your meter, insulin or medication, just keep drinking plenty of sugar-free liquids. Your blood sugar will probably go very high, but some of the sugar will spill into your urine. By drinking plenty of liquids, you can prevent dehydration and help your kidneys lower the blood sugar a little bit at a time.

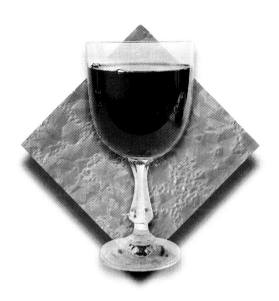

Chapter 22:   Alcohol and Diabetes

Eat, drink, and be merry. Ahhhh... if only it were that simple.

Eat too much, and you get high blood sugar and start gaining weight. Act too merry, and nobody takes you seriously. Before you know it, the men with white suits and strait jackets will be looking for you. And as far as drinking goes, you had better be careful: the only thing more dangerous than having low blood sugar is having low blood sugar when you (and everyone else) thinks you are just a bumbling drunk.

First, the good news.

For most people with diabetes, it is OK to drink small amounts of alcohol from time to time. There is no reason to avoid a glass of wine on Holidays; a champagne toast at celebrations; even a beer with your buddies. Believe it or not, research has shown that small amounts of alcohol can have beneficial effects on the heart by increasing HDL ("good" cholesterol) levels and helping you to relax.

The keys to safe drinking are to: (1) limit your alcohol intake so that you do not become intoxicated, and (2) consider alcoholic drinks as foods that can, and do, affect blood sugar levels.

Because it contains calories (6 per gram), alcohol can cause weight gain. Some drinks, such as wine, wine coolers, beer, frozen drinks and mixed drinks with fruit juice contain carbohydrates that can raise the blood sugar level. If you are counting exchanges, a single "serving" of alcohol (12 ounces beer, 4 ounces wine, 1.5 ounces hard liquor) should count as two fat exchanges. Any carbohydrates that are contained in your drink must be accounted for when you figure your starch exchanges or total grams of carbohydrate (see below). Beware of frozen drinks and drinks that use sweet mixers because they may contain very large amounts of sugar.

DRINK TYPE	AMOUNT	GRAMS CARBOHYDRATE
Regular Beer	12 oz	14
Light Beer	12 oz	6
Gin, Vodka, Whiskey, Scotch, Burbon, Rum	1.5 oz	0
Dry Wine	4 oz	1-2
Sweet Wine	4 oz	5-10
Champagne	4 oz	4
Wine Cooler	12 oz	22
Sherry	2 oz	2
Sweet Sherry	2 oz	7
Dry Vermouth	3 oz	4
Sweet Vermouth	3 oz	14

How alcohol can cause low blood sugar

Remember, sugar in the bloodstream comes from two sources: the food you eat, and the body's liver which releases its stored-up sugar into the blood at a steady rate. Your dose of insulin or diabetes pills is designed to match the total effect of your food intake and your liver:

Carbohydrate in food + Sugar released by the liver
= Total amount of sugar in the blood

When you drink alcohol, the liver starts working to "detoxify" the body - that is, it becomes very busy dealing with the alcohol, and doesn't have time to release its normal amount of sugar into the bloodstream. As a result, it is easy to get low blood sugar when you are drinking. So the first rule of drinking is this:

> **Never drink on an empty stomach. Snack on moderate amounts of carbohydrate-containing food, such as pretzels or popcorn, when drinking.**

Other hazards

For a moment, put yourself in the place of another person. If you see a person with low blood sugar, how do they act? A little bit strange, perhaps? Probably has poor coordination, slurred speech, and isn't making much sense.

Now imagine yourself at a party, where everyone is drinking and carrying on. How are they acting? A little strange perhaps? Probably have poor coordination, slurred speech, and aren't making much sense. In other words, a person in this crowd could have low blood sugar and nobody would know it. Many people with low blood sugar have been arrested for public drunkenness after having just one or two drinks simply because of the smell of alcohol on their breath.

> If you choose to drink alcohol, do so in moderation and make sure you have a companion/partner with you that knows how to respond if you have symptoms of low blood sugar. Wear medical identification at all times.

The most common time for severe low blood sugar after drinking is the middle of the night while you sleep. This is when the liver usually releases a great deal of sugar into the bloodstream. If the liver is busy dealing with alcohol, it will not be maintaining your blood sugar level.

> If you choose to drink, do so early in the evening and have a big bedtime snack.

Make sure your partner is aware that glucagon will not work if you have severe low blood sugar and have been drinking. Glucagon usually works by getting the liver to release extra sugar into the blood. However, if the liver is busy dealing with alcohol, it will not respond to glucagon. If you lose consciousness due to low blood sugar, you will need intravenous glucose from emergency paramedics.

It is best to avoid alcohol entirely after exercising. The combined effect of exercise (making the body more sensitive to insulin) and alcohol (keeping the liver from releasing its normal amount of sugar) can cause low blood sugar several hours after exercise.

Besides putting you at risk for low blood sugar, alcohol carries other harmful side effects. Alcohol contains lots of calories. It also causes the body to produce triglycerides, a form of fat. People trying to lose weight will find it very difficult if they continue to drink alcohol. More than two alcohol-containing drinks a day will also raise the blood pressure. This is very dangerous for anyone with a history of heart problems or high blood pressure. Blood pressure-lowering drugs are less effective when you drink alcohol. Stroke is also more common in people who drink.

Alcohol also causes the body to lose potassium through the urine. If you are taking diuretics (water pills), alcohol consumption could cause you to have a dangerously low potassium level.

Absolute no-no's

With certain health conditions, any alcohol consumption is extremely dangerous.

If you have PANCREATITIS (inflammation of the pancreas), you are already producing less insulin than usual. Alcohol consumption makes pancreatitis even worse, causing your diabetes to become worse.

If you have NEUROPATHY (reduced nerve sensation, especially in the feet and legs), alcohol will make it worse.

If you have RETINOPATHY (damage to the blood vessels in the eye), alcohol can cause further damage or lead to a loss of vision.

If you have HIGH TRIGLYCERIDES, you are at a very high risk for circulatory problems such as heart attack, stroke, and poor blood flow to the feet and legs. Alcohol causes triglycerides to be even higher, and thus should be avoided.

If you have a HISTORY OF SEVERE LOW BLOOD SUGAR, alcohol is likely to produce a dangerous reaction.

IF YOU TAKE DIABETES PILLS or medications for other health conditions, ask you doctor or pharmacist about possible dangers of drinking alcohol.

Key point:

Always eat while you are drinking alcohol.
Never drink on an empty stomach.

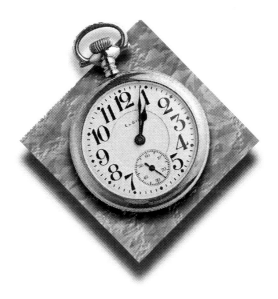

Chapter 23:   Fatigue and Diabetes

On the East side of town, Maria has just returned home from work. Is it her imagination, or do the days seem to be getting longer and longer? Used to be she had lots of energy after work. She would spend time with her kids, make a nice dinner, and still have enough left to do some exercise while watching TV. Now, she can barely make it through the front door before she plops down in an exhausted heap. What used to come easy now takes a great deal of effort, and if there's one thing Maria doesn't have, it's energy to spare.

On the West side of town, Reggie is snoozing away on the sofa with the TV on. Geraldo just uncovered another UFO conspiracy, but Reggie is oblivious to it. When he first retired, Reggie was hardly ever home. If he wasn't out on the golf course, he would be at the community center playing bridge or doing volunteer work with local kids. These days, all Reggie seems to do is stay home, watching TV and falling asleep.

Maria and Reggie are both victims of diabetes-related fatigue - chronic tiredness and lack of energy. Fatigue is not normal, and it is not healthy. It keeps you from taking care of yourself and enjoying the good things in life. If you find yourself dragging a great deal, don't just attribute it to "aging," because aging by itself should not cause you to feel fatigued. There is usually an underlying cause for fatigue, and finding the cause is the first step to correcting it.

Fatigue Factors

Although diabetes itself is not a cause of fatigue, many of the conditions associated with diabetes can cause chronic fatigue:

Hyperglycemia - If your blood sugar has been above normal or has been on the rise for a while, you may not notice any dramatic changes in your health. The changes are so slow and gradual that they "sneak up" on you. One of the side effects is fatigue. When blood sugar levels are high, your cells are not receiving all the energy they need. As a result, your body tends to run down easily.

High blood sugar also causes a sense of sleepiness. Even in people who do not have diabetes, it is common to feel sleepy after a big meal.

If your blood sugar levels are above 140 before meals or above 180 after meals, you are susceptible to fatigue. An HbA1c value greater than 8 also correlates with chronically high blood sugars and a tendency to feel fatigued. Bringing your blood sugar levels down towards normal will help you feel more energetic.

<u>Hypoglycemia</u>: If high blood sugar causes fatigue, then low blood sugar must give you more energy, right? Wrong. Low blood sugar is physically and emotionally draining. The body expends a great deal of energy trying to warn you when your blood sugar is low (shaking, sweating, etc.) and raise the blood sugar. The adrenaline surge you get during low blood sugar is usually followed by a lull in the body's metabolism.

Frequent low blood sugars put your body through a great deal of stress that can leave you feeling drained. Reducing the frequency and severity of your low blood sugars can help improve your overall energy level. See chapter 14 for tips on preventing hypoglycemia.

<u>Hypothyroidism</u>: The thyroid gland is located just below the Adam's Apple in the neck. It produces thyroid hormone, a substance that regulates the body's metabolism. When thyroid hormone levels are normal, the body tends to burn calories efficiently and have more than enough energy for daily living. When thyroid hormone levels are low, the body's metabolism can drop very low. Not only can this lead to weight gain (since the body is slow to burn calories), but it can also lead to fatigue.

It is very common for people with diabetes to develop an under-active thyroid. The same auto-immune process that attacks the pancreas and keeps it from producing enough insulin can also attack the thyroid gland and keep it from producing enough thyroid hormone.

TSH (THYROID STIMULATING HORMONE)

TSH is chemical in the blood that "tickles" the thyroid gland to produce more thyroid hormone. When the level of thyroid hormone in the blood is low, the pituitary gland produces TSH. If the TSH level is very high, it usually means that the thyroid gland is unable to make enough thyroid hormone.

Your doctor can order a lab test called a "TSH" (thyroid stimulating hormone) to see if your thyroid is functioning properly. If you are not producing enough thyroid hormone, you will probably need to take a pill (Synthroid) to increase your thyroid level. Synthroid is very effective for increasing the metabolism and restoring energy, and has virtually no side effects at the proper doses.

Depression: As described in detail in Chapter 18, depression is very common in people with diabetes. The symptoms of depression include difficulty sleeping, an inability to concentrate, uncontrollable negative thoughts, and chronic aches and pains – all of which contribute to fatigue.

Remember, depression does not necessarily mean that you cry a lot, and it is not something that you bring on yourself. Depression usually involves a chemical imbalance in the brain and nervous system. This imbalance can be treated with therapies such as anti-depressant medication, psychotherapy, or even exercise.

Circulatory Problems: With diabetes comes an accelerated rate of atherosclerosis (narrowing of the arteries). People with diabetes tend to develop heart problems and poor circulation in the legs at an earlier age than most people. If the circulation is poor, the heart and other muscles will not receive adequate amounts of oxygen and nutrients. This can lead to tiredness and shortness of breath even after minor amounts of exertion such as climbing a flight of stairs or walking to a store.

This sense of tiredness, fatigue and shortness of breath could actually save your life. Many people with diabetes do not experience chest pains during a heart attack or congestive heart failure because the nerves that carry pain signals from the heart to the brain are not operating properly. Fatigue may be the only signal to warn you that there is a problem with the circulation to your heart.

Your doctor can diagnose circulatory problems through a stress test or by checking the pulses in your legs. If you have a circulatory problem, treatment may be as simple as performing certain exercises or taking a medication to dilate your blood vessels. In serious cases, surgery may be required. Regardless of the treatment, it is very important to have the problem corrected before a critical situation arises.

Poor Diet: If your diet is lacking in certain vitamins or minerals, your body may not be able to perform at an optimal level. This can result in frequent illnesses, slow recovery from injuries, and fatigue. A dietitian at your local hospital can assess your diet to see if you are deficient in any areas. Taking a daily multiple vitamin/mineral supplement might also be helpful.

Inactivity: Remember the saying, "Use it, or lose it." Unfortunately, this statement can be very true. If you get very little exercise, your body responds in some negative ways:

- your metabolism slows down, leading to weight gain

- you become less sensitive to insulin, leading to higher blood sugar levels

- your muscles tend to become smaller and weaker

- your circulation becomes diminished

All of these changes are harmful to your health, and all can lead to fatigue. Regular exercise can not only improve your energy level throughout the day, but it is also a great way to maintain your energy level and keep it from fading as you age.

Stop the cycle!

Diabetes and fatigue are like partners in crime. Each one makes the other a little bit worse. Diabetes, especially when blood sugar levels are not well-controlled, can cause fatigue. Fatigue, in turn, can make us less likely to monitor our blood sugar, exercise and eat right. As control worsens, fatigue worsens as well.

Feelings of tiredness and lethargy should not be ignored and attributed to "old age" or "poor health". Find the cause of your fatigue and fix it. You'll be amazed at what you've been missing!

Key point:

**Fatigue is a common "side effect" of diabetes,
but it is preventable and treatable.**

Section V

Preventing and Treating Complications

Remember when you were a kid: Licking an ice cream cone in the park on a warm summer day; getting big wads of cotton candy on your face at a carnival; gulping down a box of Cracker Jacks at a baseball game. Yep, life was sweet. Who would have thought that sugar could be a source of so many problems later in life?

Actually, the sugar in your diet has little to do with the complications of diabetes. It is the extra sugar in your bloodstream that tends to cause trouble. Over a period of many years, extra sugar in the blood gradually causes damage to many of the body's organs and systems. It does this by sticking to things in the blood and changing the way they work. Sugar sticks to just about everything in sight - proteins, cholesterol, red blood cells, muscle, tendons, and the walls of the blood vessels themselves.

The results of long-term high blood sugar levels can be devastating: eye disease which can lead to blindness; kidney disease which may require dialysis or a kidney transplant; large blood vessel disease which can lead to heart attack, stroke and lower limb amputation; and nerve disease which can lead to impotency, digestive problems, impaired balance, and a loss of sensation in the hands, legs and feet.

Now, before you get down in the dumps, it is very important to know that the complications of diabetes are preventable and treatable if you take care of yourself. In this section, we will discuss the causes, symptoms and treatment options for the various long-term complications of diabetes. More importantly, we will focus on the steps you can take immediately to lower your risk for all the different complications, and if you already have complications, how to keep them from getting worse... and getting the better of you.

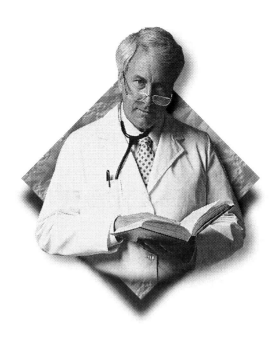

Chapter 24:   Your Health Care Team and You

Imagine that you are the coach of a baseball team. Your job depends on your team's ability to win ball games. Nothing else. You could be a brilliant coach, but if the team finishes the season 40 games out of first place, chances are that you will be spending next summer deep-sea fishing off the coast of Florida.

The question is, how do you get the team to win games? Obviously, you want to put the best team possible out on the field. You need pitchers who can throw strikes, fielders who can catch and throw, and hitters who can make contact and run the bases. If you had a billion dollars to spend, you could attract all the best free agents to your team, but this is the real world: nobody has unlimited money to spend on player salaries. So, you put together the best combination of players you can with the resources available to you.

Is your job done? Hardly. Many teams have failed to win pennants with a bunch of high-priced stars who refuse to be "team players." This is where you earn your salary. Coaching a team of baseball players means practicing fundamentals, developing strategy, and getting all your players to sacrifice personal glory for the good of the team. The players could not win without your leadership and direction, and you certainly could not win without their performance on the field.

Why all the talk about baseball? Simple. Coaching a baseball team is a lot like managing your diabetes. It takes a team effort to come out a winner.

YOU CAN NOT MANAGE YOUR DIABETES AND PREVENT LONG-TERM COMPLICATIONS WITHOUT A GOOD TEAM BEHIND YOU.

Just like a coach needs good players, you need quality health care professionals to help you do the job. But remember, even the best health professionals need "coaching" - it is your responsibility to lead them, direct them, and participate in your own care.

Your Starting Lineup

Pitching: The Physician

Your physician is the centerpiece of your health care team. He/she is ultimately responsible for diagnosing and treating your diabetes, screening for complications, prescribing the necessary tests and medications, and making sure that your control is on target.

Of course, different physicians have different levels of expertise in treating diabetes. Generally, an endocrinologist has the most experience and skill at helping people manage their diabetes. Some endocrinologists specialize in diabetes while others may treat a variety of diseases.

Internal medicine specialists (Internists) usually treat a variety of chronic health conditions, diabetes being just one of them. Some internists have a great deal of expertise in treating diabetes while others specialize in different areas.

General Practitioners (family doctors) typically treat many short-term and long-term illnesses and often have only a basic understanding of how to manage diabetes. However, any physician can provide excellent diabetes care if he calls on the resources of other health professionals (diabetes educators) to help patients with their control.

Regardless of the type of doctor you choose, you and your physician should form a partnership. Your doctor is not your boss, but rather a consultant that you have hired to help you coordinate your care. Remember, you are the person in charge of your care; not your doctor. If your doctor tries to overburden you or leave you out of the decision-making process, he is not doing a good job as a consultant.

Here are some tips for getting the most out of your partnership with your doctor:

1. Learn all you can about your diabetes. Read books and magazines. Take courses. Attend seminars. Watch educational videos. The more you know, the more confident you will become, and the better you can communicate with your doctor.

2. Take your doctor's advice. Too many people pay a consultant top dollar, and then don't do what they recommend. If your doctor

recommends that you take insulin, do it. If he suggests that you see a counselor or a specialist, it is probably in your best interest to do so.

3. Keep good, neat records and bring them to every visit. Ratty-looking napkins with numbers scrawled on them haphazardly are not going to do anybody any good. Ask your doctor about the specific information she needs and be sure to bring it with you. It is usually helpful to keep track of your blood sugar levels, carbohydrate intake, physical activities and insulin/medication doses, and record them all on the same page.

4. Prepare questions in writing for every visit. Writing them down will ensure that you don't forget to ask anything. There are no dumb questions, and it is your doctor's job as a consultant to answer your questions - so don't hesitate to ask.

5. If you do not understand what your doctor is saying, ask her to explain it in simpler terms. Many doctors are guilty of explaining things in "medical mumbo jumbo."

6. Get all of your doctor's recommendations in writing so that there is no confusion later on. Diabetes management can be very complex, so keep everything on paper and in correct order.

7. Stay on top of your lab tests and physical examinations. See your doctor at least once every three months, and take your shoes and socks off so she can examine your feet. Keep a checklist handy so that you can keep track of your lab results and physical examinations; remind your doctor of when actions need to be taken:

LAB TEST ...	SHOULD BE DONE ...
Hemoglobin Alc	Every 3 months (if you take insulin)
	Every 6 months (if not taking insulin)
Thyroid Function (TSH)	Once a year
Urine Microalbumin	Once a year
Blood Lipids (total cholesterol, HDL, LDL, triglycerides)	Once a year

EXAMINATION ...	SHOULD BE DONE ...
Foot Exam	Every Visit
Blood Pressure	Every Visit
Weight	Every Visit
Dilated Eye Exam	At Least Once A Year
Dental Exam	Twice A Year
Screening for Neuropathy	Once A Year
Pulses in Feet and Legs	Once A Year

Now here's a question: What would you do as coach of a baseball team if a pitcher is not doing the job? Chances are you would try to coach him through it by offering some suggestions. If that didn't work, or if the pitcher refused to be coached, you would probably make a trade.

IT IS YOUR RIGHT (AND RESPONSIBILITY) TO SWITCH DOCTORS IF YOU ARE NOT SATISFIED WITH THE SERVICE YOU ARE RECEIVING.

Of course, switching doctors is a measure that should be considered carefully. Continuity of care (establishing a relationship with a single doctor over a period of time) has its benefits, so your first move should be to try to fix any problems. Talk to your doctor if you are not satisfied with her service. Try to work out your differences. Most doctors are willing to do what it takes to meet your needs, and she may actually appreciate your feedback and concern.

However, if you continue to have problems with your doctor, don't hesitate to make a switch. You should consider leaving your doctor if she:

1. Does not explain things in a way you can understand

2. Won't answer your questions or spend enough time with you

3. Fails to perform the necessary screenings for diabetic complications

4. Does not order the proper lab tests in a timely manner

5. Will not recognize the importance of your cultural traditions when devising your diabetes management plan

6. Refuses to refer you to a specialist such as an endocrinologist, podiatrist or dietitian

7. For personal reasons, denies you of access to current technology such as an insulin pump or monitoring device

8. Does not recognize the importance of obtaining tight blood sugar control, or has not been successful at helping you improve your control

Catcher: The Certified Diabetes Educator

Believe it or not, 19 out of 20 people with diabetes have only their physician to turn to for assistance with their diabetes care. That would be like a baseball team with a pitcher but no fielders. If your pitcher can strike everyone out, there is no problem. But not too many pitchers can do that. You need players in the field to handle the ball once it is hit.

One of the key players on your team is a Certified Diabetes Educator (CDE). A CDE is often a nurse, but it can also be a dietitian, pharmacist, exercise physiologist, physician, mental health counselor, or anyone in the health care field with advanced training in diabetes management.

In many cases, a CDE will be able to teach you and guide you through the day-to-day management of your diabetes. Whereas a physician often has limited time to spend with you and is not trained in the fine art of teaching, a CDE will take the time to teach you how to self-manage your diabetes. Topics a CDE can teach you include:

- How to do home blood glucose monitoring

- How to make safe adjustments to your insulin or medication doses

- How to inject insulin with a syringe or pen

- Timing of meals, snacks, exercise and insulin injections

- Basic nutrition skills, such as meal planning and carbohydrate counting

- How to manage your diabetes when you get sick

- Benefits and precautions of exercise

- Prevention, detection and treatment of low blood sugar

- Proper foot care and other self-care practices for preventing complications

To locate a CDE in your area, talk to your doctor or contact the American Association of Diabetes Educators and ask for the CDE referral program (see Appendix B).

First Base: The Dietitian

As the person ultimately responsible for catching the ball and making the outs, the first baseman is involved in almost every play. Any time you check your blood sugar, what you ate and when you ate will almost always be a major factor. Working with a good dietary counselor can make the difference between good control and no control at all.

In the past, the role of the dietitian was been to give diet sheets to people with diabetes, explain the "exchange" system, and hope for the best. Inevitably, the diet sheets would find their way into the trash, the doctor provided little support, and the person with diabetes wound up confused and frustrated.

Today, a dietitian can help you design a meal plan that incorporates your choices for meals, snacks and yes, even desserts. No longer should you be given a diet sheet and told everything you should and shouldn't eat. No longer are sweets forbidden. No longer is dietary counseling a one-time visit. And no longer should your doctor act as your dietary counselor.

EVERYONE WITH DIABETES SHOULD WORK WITH
A DIETITIAN (preferably an RD, CDE)
ON AN ONGOING BASIS.

A good dietitian will assess your nutritional needs, current food habits, attitudes concerning food, lifestyle/schedule, and caloric requirements. Based on these, the dietitian will work with you to increase your knowledge of nutrition, set goals, learn new behaviors to achieve the goals, and measure your progress in achieving weight control and blood sugar management. Your partner (spouse, roommate, guardian, etc.) will play an important role in helping you design and follow your meal plan, so he/she should participate in your consultations with the dietitian.

Some specific topics a dietitian can help with include:

- How to count carbohydrates and adjust insulin doses based on carbohydrate intake.

- Safe consumption of alcohol.

- What to do for special occasions such as parties, holidays, travel and vacations.

- Reading food labels and choosing appropriate foods in the supermarket.

- Ways to stay on your meal plan when dining out.

- The role of meal timing and snacks in controlling blood sugar levels.

- Dietary strategies for lowering your cholesterol and improving your HDL and LDL levels.

- Incorporating foods for religious holidays and ethnic traditions.

Obviously, it will take more than one session to cover these topics, and more questions will probably come up along the way. Plan to visit your dietitian several times, and maintain contact every three to six months to address new dietary issues. Your dietitian is your teacher, your advisor, and your pep squad!

Second Base: The Counselor

The prototype second baseman is a steady, sure-handed individual that you can count on in the clutch. A mental health counselor offers the same kind of helping hand with your diabetes management. With all the pressure placed on people with diabetes to manage blood sugar levels while taking care of everything else in their lives, it is no wonder that issues such as these often arise:

- Denial of having diabetes

- Eating disorders

- Depression

- Insomnia

- Anger

- Compulsion/Obsession

- Difficulty with personal relationships

- Financial hardship

- Job discrimination

Imagine how difficult it would be for a baseball player (or anyone, for that matter) to do his job if his mind is preoccupied with deeper concerns about his health and well-being. It would make concentration virtually impossible, judgment poor, reflexes slow, and compliance with a complex game plan very unlikely. In other words, psychological issues must be dealt with before you can expect to do an effective job at controlling your diabetes.

If you have concerns that are interfering with you ability to take good care of yourself, don't hesitate to discuss them with a psychiatrist, psychologist or social worker.

Third Base: The Exercise Physiologist

Third base is known as the "hot corner". Exercise is a hot topic in diabetes because of all the benefits it offers people with Type-I or Type-II diabetes. However, you can also get yourself in hot water if you exercise improperly. The risks associated with exercise are numerous for people with diabetes: hypoglycemia, foot injury and bringing out underlying heart problems just to name a few.

An exercise physiologist is a health professional who understands the physical, psychological and metabolic effects of exercise. He/she can help you in the following areas:

- Designing an exercise plan, including types of activities, frequency, duration and intensity.

- Keeping you motivated

- Stretching and flexibility

- Strength training

- Adjustments for preventing low blood sugar

- Weight loss and body composition measurements (body fat reduction)

Look for an exercise physiologist with at least a Masters-level degree. Ideally, he/she should be affiliated with a hospital or diabetes treatment center. An exercise physiologist who is also a CDE may be your best option.

Shortstop: The Pharmacist

There is nobody out, with a runner on third base in the late innings of a close game. The ball is hit sharply to the left side of the infield. The shortstop makes a diving stop of the ball. He gets up, and instead of throwing to first for an easy out, he whirls around and fires a strike to home plate to nail the runner trying to score. That's pretty much the shortstop's job: to make the kind of plays and decisions that help the team win games.

Your pharmacist can do much more than just take prescriptions from your doctor and fill them. She can be a source of excellent advice and guidance for controlling your diabetes and other health conditions. Ask your pharmacist for assistance in any of these areas:

- Selecting over-the-counter medicines without sugar and alcohol

- Screening for harmful drug interactions (if you take more than one medication)

- Finding out if certain over-the-counter medicines will interact with your prescription drugs

- Learning about side effects from the drugs you are taking

- Emergency refills when traveling (via overnight mail or by calling a pharmacy near you)

- Recommending the latest (and best) over-the-counter medicines for common conditions such as headache, arthritis, menstrual cramps, upset stomach, nausea, diarrhea, urinary tract infection, dry skin and colds/congestion

- Obtaining the latest and least costly diabetes supplies

Outfielders:

The Podiatrist, The Ophthalmologist and The Dentist

A smart baseball coach will fill his outfield with specialists: The left fielder is usually a power hitter capable of driving in lots of runs. Center field is best covered by a speedy sort who can track down long fly balls and steal a few bases. The right fielder had better have a cannon for an arm so that he can throw out base runners trying to score from second or third.

Your diabetes team's outfield should be filled with top-notch health specialists who you can call on periodically to help prevent and treat the long-term complications of diabetes. These are people who are on the periphery of your team - they will not be involved in your day-to-day blood sugar management, but they are essential nonetheless.

A podiatrist plays a key role in treating foot problems before they become serious. Rather than self-treating minor foot ailments and ignoring deformities, have them evaluated and treated by a podiatrist as quickly as possible. The role of the podiatrist will be covered in detail in Chapter 30.

Timely eye care is essential for preserving your vision. As we will discuss in Chapter 27, diabetic eye disease (retinopathy) can be treated successfully if caught early. There are usually no symptoms associated with retinopathy until it is quite advanced. If it is allowed to progress to an advanced stage before you seek treatment, you may lose your vision entirely.

Have your eyes examined at least once a year by an OPHTHAL-MOLOGIST. This is a medical doctor who is skilled at detecting and treating diabetic retinopathy. Your eye exam should include drops in your eyes (to dilate the pupils) and use of a bright light to inspect the tiny blood vessels in the back of the eye. Simply having your doctor check your eyes quickly during an office visit is not sufficient to detect retinopathy.

Finally, consider your dentist part of your diabetes team. People with diabetes have a tendency to develop gum disease earlier and more severely than people without diabetes. See your dentist at least twice a year for a thorough gum exam and cleaning (removal of plaque). Add your own daily brushing and flossing and you should have plenty to smile about!

Key point:

Make it your responsibility to see the members of your health care team, obtain lab tests, and receive examinations in a timely manner.

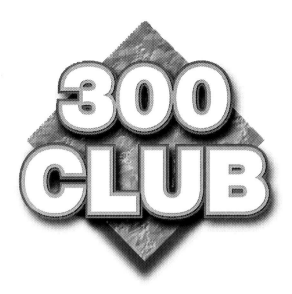

Chapter 25: Welcome to the 300 Club!

As Groucho Marx used to say, "I wouldn't want to belong to any club that would have me as a member." The "300 Club" is one of those clubs where you would be well served to take Groucho's advice.

The "300 Club refers to a set of potentially harmful health conditions. These include high blood pressure, high cholesterol, high triglycerides, high blood sugar, and excess body weight. Often, the total cholesterol, triglycerides, blood sugar and weight are in the 300s - thus the name, the 300 Club.

It is very common for a person who is overweight to also have high blood sugar, high blood pressure and elevated blood lipids. Since they occur together so often, scientists believe that there is a common thread that runs through all of these conditions. The problems are referred to collectively as "Syndrome X" because the underlying cause is still unknown. Perhaps there is a single gene, chemical imbalance, or biological reaction that triggers them. Whatever the cause, Syndrome X is a mean and destructive force that can lead to severe health problems.

The harmful effects of Syndrome X

Betty is a typical victim of Syndrome X. You might say that she has been a lifetime member of the 300 Club. She is overweight, tipping the scales at 234 pounds. She has had Type-II diabetes for many years. Her HbA1c test indicates poor control - average blood sugars of close to 330. She takes medication to control her blood pressure, and was warned by her doctor to cut the fat in her diet because her cholesterol level is way too high. Betty is also tired and hungry most of the time.

A few months ago, Betty had to undergo surgery to treat an infection in her foot. The circulation in her legs had become so bad that nothing would heal on its own. To make matters worse, she suffered a mild heart attack soon after returning home. Today, Betty is bedridden and requires a visiting nurse to take care of her.

Syndrome X exerts its most damaging effects on the circulation. Obesity, hypertension, hyperglycemia, high cholesterol and high triglycerides all impair the flow of blood throughout the body. They cause narrowing, constriction and hardening of the arteries, meaning that vital organs may not be receiving enough oxygen and nutrients. This can lead to stroke, heart attack, muscle pain, poor healing of wounds, cold extremities, and a general sense of weakness.

High blood sugar (hyperglycemia)

Elevated blood sugar levels are a major cause of circulatory problems. Imagine trying to run thick maple syrup through a very narrow pipe, and you should get an idea of the effect high blood sugar can have on blood flow.

The DCCT (Diabetes Control and Complications Trial) proved that lowering blood sugar levels will reduce the risk of the complications of diabetes (see Chapter 9). Your long-term goal should be to get your readings as close to normal as possible throughout the day and night. However, if your blood sugar levels are running very high now, your immediate goal should be to lower them just a little bit. Perhaps you could make some changes in your diet, start exercising, monitor your blood sugar more frequently, or make changes to your insulin or medication. Remember, every little improvement counts!

Obesity (overweight)

Excess body fat places a strain on the heart and blood vessels by forcing them to work even harder than usual. You not only have to delivery adequate blood flow to your body's muscles and organs, but now you have to nourish all those fat cells throughout your body. Excess body fat also contributes to large amounts of triglycerides in the blood, which as we will discuss, causes further problems with the circulation.

We all know about the benefits of permanent weight loss. However, nothing can help you beat Syndrome X better than ridding your body of excess fat. By losing as little as 20 pounds, you may see significant improvements in your blood pressure, blood sugar and cholesterol levels. For tips on safe and effective weight loss, see Chapter 16.

Blood lipids

"Blood lipids" refers to a variety of different fats and cholesterol in the bloodstream.

"HDLs" (high density lipoproteins) are globs of fat and protein (mostly protein) that circulate in the bloodstream. HDLs actually remove cholesterol from the walls of blood vessels and carry them back to the liver for processing. HDLs are referred to as "good cholesterol" because they lower the risk of heart disease and circulatory problems. YOU WANT YOUR HDL LEVEL TO BE AS HIGH AS POSSIBLE.

"LDSs" (low density lipoproteins) and "VLDLs" (very low density lipoproteins) are also made up of a combination of fat and protein, but have less protein and more fat than HDLs. LDLs and VLDLs are mean critters - they circulate in the bloodstream and deposit fat in the walls of blood vessels, resulting in plaques and narrowing of the arteries. YOU WANT YOUR LDLs AND VLDLs TO BE AS LOW AS POSSIBLE.

LDL should be below 130 in most people with diabetes, and below 100 in people who are already at a high risk for circulatory problems due to obesity, high blood pressure, or a family (or personal) history of heart attack/stroke.

Total Cholesterol is a sum total of HDLs, LDLs, and VLDLs. A high cholesterol level usually means that there are a lot of LDLs and VLDLs messing things up in the bloodstream, so keeping total cholesterol under 200 is very important. However, it is more important to achieve a healthy relationship between HDLs and LDLs. Each HDL has the power to halt the effects of about 31/2 LDLs, so your goal should be to have no more than 31/2 times as many LDLs as HDLs.

Triglycerides are giant molecules of fat that are packed into the body's fat cells. Some triglycerides also circulate in the bloodstream to be used for energy. High levels of triglycerides can cause problems, especially for people with diabetes. Research has shown that triglycerides keep insulin from doing its job of lowering blood sugar levels. That is, they cause "insulin resistance". Triglycerides also cause LDLs to become more potent, which leads to more narrowing and hardening of the arteries. YOU WANT YOUR TRIGLYCERIDES TO BE AS LOW AS POSSIBLE. A goal for most people with diabetes should be to keep triglycerides below 200.

Lowering them lipids

Have your doctor order lab tests for a complete lipid panel every year. You will need to have the test done first thing in the morning after an overnight fast (nothing to eat since the night before) in order to obtain accurate HDL and LDL readings. Remember, a total cholesterol level only gives part of the picture - it does not tell us anything about the important relationship between HDLs and LDLs. So make sure to have a complete set of lipid measurements.

To summarize, your blood lipid goals should be as follows:

Total Cholesterol	<200
HDL	>35
LDL	<130 <100 (high risk)
Triglycerides	<200
Total Chol./HDL Ratio	<5 (males) <4.4 (females)
LDL/HDL Ratio	<3.5 (males) <3.2 (females)

People with diabetes may have a more difficult time than most people in lowering triglyceride levels. Insulin resistance (caused by obesity) causes the liver to make extra triglycerides. A diet low in fat and high in carbohydrates can help reduce cholesterol levels, but it may have the opposite effect on triglycerides. For these reasons, it is best to work with a dietitian when trying to lower cholesterol and triglyceride levels at the same time.

Essentially, you have five tools as your disposal for improving your blood lipids:

1. Exercise - Low-impact aerobic exercises such as walking, swimming and bicycling are effective ways to lower triglycerides and total cholesterol. They can also help maintain or raise HDLs, which protect us from heart disease.

2. Dietary Changes - Changing your diet is another effective way to lower your cholesterol and triglyceride levels. The most helpful change you can make is to reduce the amount of fat you eat. The more fat you eat, the more LDLs and fewer HDLs your liver will produce. Some specific dietary changes you can make include:

   • Eating fewer high-cholesterol foods such as egg yolks, dairy foods (whole milk, cheese), organ meats (liver, kidney, brain) and animal meats (beef, poultry). But remember, of the cholesterol that circulates in your blood, only 30% comes from what you eat. The rest comes from the liver, so cutting your dietary cholesterol alone will not get the job done completely.

   • Cutting down on foods high in saturated fat such as red meat, butter, cheese, whole milk, coconut oil and palm oil. Saturated fats cause the liver to pump out more LDL cholesterol.

- When choosing fats, look for monounsaturated fat. This type of fat can actually raise HDLs without increasing triglycerides. Foods rich in monounsaturated fat include olive oil, canola oil, nuts, avocados and fish.

- Have more soluble fiber (oats, beans, fruit). Fiber keeps cholesterol in the diet from being absorbed into the bloodstream.

- Drink less caffeine and alcohol. Both of these raise the level of triglycerides in the blood.

3. If you smoke, quit smoking. Cigarette smoking suppresses production of HDLs and greatly increases your risk for circulatory problems.

4. Control your blood sugar levels. Aggressive blood sugar control usually leads to a reduction in both cholesterol and triglycerides. For individuals with Type-II diabetes, Metformin (Glucophage) has been shown to have beneficial effects on blood lipids.

5. Take advantage of cholesterol-lowering medications. These include:

- Nicotinic Acid/Niacin - Lowers cholesterol and triglycerides and increases HDL, but often causes blood sugar levels to rise (this limits its use in people with diabetes). Available over-the-counter; start with a small dose and increase it gradually.

- Gemfibrozil (Lopid) - Medication of choice for lowering very high triglyceride and cholesterol levels. May take 3-6 months to start seeing an effect.

- Reductase Inhibitors (Mevacor, Zocor, Pravachol, Lescol) - Lower the production of cholesterol by the liver. Good for lowering moderately high LDLs and triglycerides, especially in people with diabetes.

- Cholestyramine (Questran) - Forces the liver to take cholesterol out of the blood by binding with bile salts. Works best when cholesterol is high but triglycerides are normal.

- Estrogen - Should be used by women during or after menopause to lower LDL and increase HDL as well as prevent osteoporosis.

- Antioxidant (Vitamin E) - 400 to 800 units of Vitamin E daily can help prevent the damaging effects of LDL cholesterol.

The pressure's on

One out of five Americans has high blood pressure (hypertension). Like diabetes, hypertension is a life-long disease that affects many parts of the body. High blood pressure is very common in people with Type-II diabetes. Blood pressure is normal in people with Type-I diabetes. Kidney damage in Type-I diabetes casues high blood pressure.

BLOOD PRESSURE

The amount of force exerted on the walls of blood vessels as blood flows through. Pressure that is too high can cause damage to blood vessels.

With Syndrome X, high blood pressure can occur long before kidney disease develops. Hypertension may be related to obesity, insulin resistance, high salt intake, caffeine consumption, and a lack of magnesium in the diet. Whatever the cause, high blood pressure causes damage to blood vessels.

> **SYSTOLIC BLOOD PRESSURE**
>
> Pressure within blood vessels when the heart is contracting (pushing blood through).
>
> **DIASTOLIC BLOOD PRESSURE**
>
> Pressure within blood vessels when the heart is relaxing (not pushing blood through).

"Normal" blood pressure is considered to be 140/90 or less. By definition, high blood pressure means a systolic number (the first number) over 140, or a diastolic number (the second number) over 90. More than 50% of all people who have had Type-II diabetes for more than 10 years have high blood pressure, and most people with Type-I diabetes who have kidney damage will have high blood pressure as well.

Keeping the blood pressure under control is critical to one's health. High blood pressure usually leads to enlargement of the heart, weakness of the heart muscle and hardening of the arteries - all of which can lead to congestive heart failure. High blood pressure can cause hardening or rupture of blood vessels leading to the brain, causing part of the brain to die due to inadequate blood flow (stroke). It also contributes to kidney failure by placing excess strain on the kidneys.

Releasing pressure

Unfortunately, the human body does not come equipped with a "release valve" in case the blood pressure becomes too high. However, there are a number of lifestyle and medical treatments that are very effective at lowering the blood pressure and keeping it in a safe range.

1. Exercise - Aerobic activity such as walking, swimming, cycling or playing tennis lowers blood pressure whether or not you lose weight. It is important to note that resistance exercise (weight lifting) does not lower blood pressure, and may be dangerous for people with uncontrolled high blood pressure.

2. Dietary Change - Limiting salt intake to no more than 3-5 grams a day (3000-5000 mg) can help lower blood pressure. A diet low in fat and calories can also lower blood pressure by helping get your weight under control. Minimizing alcohol consumption will also help, as alcohol tends to raise the blood pressure and reduce the effectiveness of blood pressure medications. Finally, reducing caffeine intake by using decaffeinated beverages can alleviate blood pressure in many cases.

3. Stop Smoking - The nicotine in tobacco causes blood vessels to constrict and stay constricted for up to several hours. Quitting smoking will allow you to take a major step toward controlling your blood pressure.

4. Self-Monitoring of Blood Pressure - Checking your blood pressure is just as important as checking your blood sugar. High blood pressure is a life-long, 24-hour disease. Daily blood pressure checks at various times of day will let you know if your current method of blood pressure control is working. Remember, a systolic reading over 140 or a diastolic reading over 90 is a sign of trouble.

By checking your own blood pressure, you can learn the effect of different foods (including salt), stress and exercise on your blood pressure, and share the results with your doctor. It can also allow you to fine-tune your blood pressure control if you become ill (dehydration lowers blood pressure), take an antidepressant medication (which may lower blood pressure), or are subject to stress at work or home (the adrenaline rush raises blood pressure temporarily).

Just as a single blood sugar test in the doctor's office is insufficient to assess your overall blood sugar control, a single blood pressure test is insufficient to evaluate your blood pressure control. In fact, many people experience "white coat syndrome" - a rise in blood pressure just from being in the strange surroundings of a doctor's office. Home monitoring will give a more accurate and reliable measurement of your true blood pressure, assuming that it is done correctly.

5. Blood Pressure Medications - A number of effective medications are available for lowering blood pressure:

- Diuretics (water pills) are drugs that lower blood pressure by causing the body to urinate away extra fluids. They tend to worsen diabetes control, increase cholesterol and triglycerides, and cause low potassium and magnesium levels.

- Beta Blockers (Propranolol, Atenolol, Nadolol, Metoprolol) are drugs that lower the blood pressure by slowing the heart rate. Beta blockers tend to increase triglycerides and lower HDLs. They can also mask symptoms of low blood sugar, since the heart rate does not increase the way it normally would when the blood sugar is low.

- Alpha Blockers (Prazosin, Terazosin, Doxazosin) relax many of the blood vessels. However, they can cause abnormally low blood pressure when a person stands up from a lying or a sitting position (especially in the elderly). The result can be dizziness, falls, and injuries.

- ACE Inhibitors are the first choice for treating high blood pressure in people with diabetes. In those with Type-I diabetes, these drugs should be started at the earliest rise in blood pressure or leakage of protein into the urine.

ACE inhibitors offer a unique combination of benefits: They slow/stop the progression of kidney damage and lower blood pressure. They may also make liver and fat cells more sensitive to insulin, so blood sugar control may improve. ACE inhibitors do not raise cholesterol levels or worsen control of diabetes. Examples include Captopril (Capoten), Accupril, Lisinopril (Zestril), and Enalpril (Vasotec).

• Calcium Channel Blockers, like ACE inhibitors, lower the blood pressure and relieve the pressure on the kidneys. They can be used in addition to or in place of ACE inhibitors. Calcium channel blockers are the drugs of choice for treating supine hypertension (blood pressure that is high when lying down but drops suddenly when sitting or standing up).

Some calcium channel blockers (Cardizem, Procardia) also improve blood flow to heart muscle. Long-acting versions of the drug (Procardia XL, Cardizem CD, Calan SR) are preferred because they have an even, steady effect and are not likely to cause blood pressure to drop too low. Calcium channel blockers do not raise cholesterol levels or affect diabetes control.

Key point:

High cholesterol, triglycerides, weight and blood pressure often occur in people with diabetes. Controlling these is essential for preventing serious health problems.

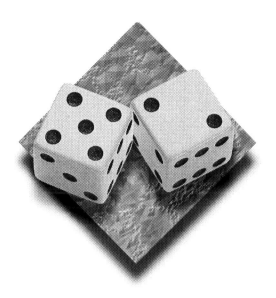

Chapter 26:   Diabetes and Kidney Damage

The kidneys, without a doubt, are the Rodney Dangerfields of bodily organs. They just don't get no respect.

The kidneys aren't much to behold. They are bean-shaped organs (we have two of them) about the size of a dinner roll, located near the lower back just above the bladder. All they do is rid the entire blood system of impurities - no small task considering all the waste products our bodies produce. In simple terms, the kidneys are the body's filters - they keep the good stuff in, and let the bad stuff flow out (through the urine). Without this filtering process, the bloodstream would become so polluted that it would kill us within a matter of hours.

Diabetes does damage

Kidney disease, also called "nephropathy", is one of the most deadly and costly complications of diabetes. In fact, diabetes is the leading cause of new cases of kidney failure in the United States.

After having diabetes for 15 years, one out of every three people with Type-I diabetes and one out of every five people with Type-II diabetes has some degree of kidney damage. Kidney disease can happen to anyone with diabetes, but it is more common in those with a family history of high blood pressure. Among people with Type-II diabetes, ethnic minorities are hit the hardest. Asian-Americans, African-Americans and Hispanic-Americans have a higher risk of kidney disease than Caucasians.

The incidence of kidney disease is on the rise in the U.S. due to the increase in Type-II diabetes. Already, $1.5 billion is spent annually to treat kidney failure, and many people who are on dialysis are unable to hold jobs. The result is a tremendous financial burden that must be met by society.

Diabetes damages the kidneys in two ways:

First, high blood sugar levels tend to make tiny blood vessels (capillaries) very fragile. Over a period of many years, these fragile capillaries may become swollen and leaky, or they may stop carrying blood altogether. The kidneys are packed full of tiny capillaries that are susceptible to damage if blood sugar levels are elevated. The kidneys also contain millions of little filters that are nourished by these capillaries. If the blood flow is impaired, the filters may start to whither away or become "leaky" (letting stuff we need, like protein, escape into the urine).

Second, diabetes often contributes to clogging of large blood vessels and elevated blood pressure. With high blood pressure, the kidney's filters are forced to work extra hard, and many will become damaged prematurely.

Don't forget, the better you control your blood sugar, the lower your risk for kidney disease. The DCCT (Diabetes Control and Complications Trial) has proven that intensive blood sugar control reduces damage to the kidneys as well as the eyes and nerves.

The stages of kidney disease

Kidney disease is not something that happens overnight. It usually takes years for kidney disease to become life-threatening. This is good, because we know how to detect and treat kidney disease in its earliest stages so that it is not likely to progress to the more harmful and serious stages.

Healthy Filter: Prior to the development of kidney damage, the kidneys do an effective job of ridding the bloodstream of impurities and waste products, and helping to retain the things we want to keep in the bloodstream such as protein. The kidneys also help to keep the blood pressure under control by keeping certain chemicals in the blood maintained at a proper level.

Hyper Filter: When blood sugar levels rise (with the development of diabetes), the kidneys are forced to work harder as more sugar and water pass through into the urine. Excessive protein in the diet can also make the kidney filters work harder. The heavy load placed on the kidneys may start causing damage to the kidney's filtration system.

Holey Filter: As time goes on and blood sugars remain high, the blood supply within the kidneys becomes damaged. Tiny holes appear in the filters, and they begin to leak small amounts of Albumin (a protein) into the urine. Blood pressure may begin to rise due to uncontrolled diabetes and the kidneys' inability to regulate blood pressure effectively.

This is the stage at which kidney damage can be detected and reversed. Any rise in blood pressure is a sign that problems may be a-brewing. Also, your doctor should ask you to perform a 24-hour urine collection each year to measure the amount of Albumin in the urine. Less than 30 mg in 24 hours indicates no sign of kidney disease. 30-300 mg in 24 hours is called microalbuminuria, and is a clear indication that kidney damage has begun. Now is the time to apply the treatments and interventions described in the next section.

Helpless Filter: When you start spilling more than 300 mg of Albumin into the urine in a single day, your kidney disease is quite advanced. At this point, your kidneys are unable to remove all the impurities from your blood. Your BUN (Blood Urea Nitrogen) will probably be high due to an excess of urea (a waste product) in the blood. Your Creatinine Clearance will probably be low, because your kidneys are not clearing (removing) the blood of enough harmful waste products. In addition, the blood pressure will continue to rise due to the kidneys' inability to achieve sodium balance in the bloodstream.

At this point, it is difficult to halt the progression of kidney disease. Protein restriction is imposed in the diet, and every effort is made to control blood pressure. Still, within five years, chances are that your kidneys will fail completely, and kidney transplantation or hemodialysis (a machine which cleanses the blood three times a week) will be necessary. Since kidney failure usually leads to additional medical problems, 50% of people placed on dialysis will die within three years.

Let's do something about it. Now.

The worst thing you can do is assume that because you have diabetes, you are destined to go into kidney failure and die. Nothing could be further from the truth. There is a lot you can do to keep your kidneys healthy and prevent small problems from becoming big ones.

Blood sugar control is your first and best line of defense against kidney damage. Research has shown that kidney damage tends to occur when the HbA1c is above 8% (average blood sugar over 180). Every effort should be made to improve your blood sugar control so that your HbA1c is below this level. This may involve checking your blood sugar more frequently and learning to adjust your insulin doses based on your physical activities and carbohydrate intake. Or, it might involve losing weight so that your insulin will work better.

Keeping your blood pressure under control is another way to prevent or reverse kidney problems. A variety of methods are available to keep your blood pressure under control (see Chapter 25 for details). Your goal should be to keep your blood pressure under 140/90. 130/70 is a realistic target for most people whose blood pressure is elevated.

ACE inhibitors and, to a lesser extent, Calcium Channel Blockers are the drugs of choice for controlling high blood pressure in people with diabetes. These medications serve a double purpose by also helping to protect the kidneys from further damage. In many cases, ACE inhibitors can actually stop or reverse the leakage of protein into the urine. Of course, you should also make every attempt to exercise, control your weight and limit your fat and salt intake, as these will also help to control your blood pressure.

Window of opportunity

Early detection of kidney problems is an important step toward preventing more serious kidney disease. Catching kidney damage at the stage of microalbuminuria (the holey filter) means that there is still time to do something about it. You should have your 24-hour urine tested for protein (Albumin) every year. People with Type-I diabetes can start the test five years after their initial diagnosis; those with Type-II diabetes should be tested every year after their initial diagnosis.

State of Kidneys	Amount of Protein Leaking into Urine	Notes
Healthy Kidneys	<30 mg/day	Keep blood pressure controlled!
Microalbuminuria	30-300 mg/day	Still reversible: Start treatment now!
Clinical Albuminuria	>300 mg/day	Difficult to treat. Will probably lead to kidney failure.

For an accurate measurement of the protein in your urine, a laboratory test is required. Microalbuminuria can be detected (but not measured accurately) in the physician's office with a special dipstick called MICRAL. Traditional dipsticks will only detect large amounts of protein, which indicates advanced kidney disease (the helpless filter stage). While microalbuminuria can be reversed, clinical proteinuria (more than 300 mg protein lost through the urine in 24 hours) is irreversible.

At the first signs of microalbuminuria, the following steps should be taken:

1. Blood glucose control should be intensified.

2. ACE inhibitors should be started to ease blood pressure, especially within the kidneys.

3. Protein in the diet should be reduced to no more than 10% of

total calories. Divide your total daily calories by 40 to arrive at your maximum grams of protein per day. Reducing the protein in the diet lessens the workload placed on the kidneys and allows them to recover.

4. All smoking must be stopped. As mentioned earlier in this chapter, smoking raises blood pressure and accelerates kidney damage.

Other things to know about kidney disease...

In many cases, kidney damage and eye damage (retinopathy) occur simultaneously. If you develop problems with one, be sure to have the other checked as soon as possible.

Certain anti-inflammatory drugs (Ibuprofen, Naprosyn) have the potential to cause kidney damage if taken on a regular basis. If you must take these drugs, be sure to have your kidney function tested frequently.

Urinary tract infections should be treated promptly due to the risk of infecting the kidneys. In addition, avoid consuming large amounts of foods high in phosphorous, such as milk and dairy products. Excess phosphorous can cause indirect damage to the kidneys.

Finally, you should be aware that rigorous exercise can raise the amount of protein excreted by the kidney for several hours after the activity. This is not a sign of kidney disease, and exercise does not damage the kidneys. However, for the sake of obtaining accurate test results, it is best to avoid vigorous exercise for 8-12 hours prior to having the urine tested for protein.

Key point:

An annual test for microalbumin (small amounts of protein in the urine) can detect kidney damage while it is still treatable and reversible.

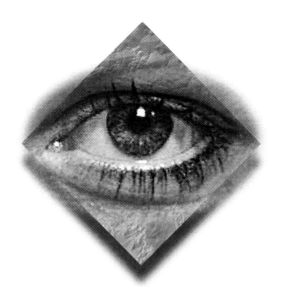

Chapter 27: Diabetes and Eye Disease

Diabetes is the leading cause of blindness in the U.S. People with diabetes are 25 times more likely than people without diabetes to experience vision loss. After 25 years of having diabetes, four out of five people will have some degree of eye damage.

Enough said. The American Diabetes Association would not adopt "Don't Be Blind to Diabetes" as its theme if eye disease was not a serious problem. But rather than dwell on the negative, this chapter will focus on the things you can do here and now to keep your eyes healthy and preserve your vision for a lifetime.

What is diabetic eye disease, and what causes it?

The first step toward taking care of your eyes is understanding a little bit about the eye and how eye damage occurs.

Think of the eye as a hollow ball with an opening (the pupil) that lets light inside. The light shines inside the ball and hits the back portion, like the way light hits film in a camera. The back of the eye where the light hits is called the "retina". The retina is a very sensitive area that needs a lot of tiny blood vessels (capillaries) to keep it healthy. The part of the retina that is responsible for most of our sharp vision is called the "macula".

You may recall from the chapter on kidney disease that high blood sugar levels can cause damage to tiny blood vessels. Capillaries may become brittle or weak, and can rupture, leak, or stop carrying nutrient-rich blood to the retina when it becomes damaged by elevated blood sugar levels.

Usually, it takes several years for damage to occur. That's why everyone with Type-I diabetes should start seeing an ophthalmologist for an eye exam every year starting five years after they are diagnosed. People with Type-II diabetes should see an ophthalmologist immediately after they are diagnosed because the diabetes may have been present for several years prior to diagnosis.

Stages of diabetic eye disease

The common term for diabetic eye disease is "retinopathy", which means "disease of the retina". Retinopathy can occur in a variety of degrees, from mild to very severe.

Background Retinopathy is the earliest form of diabetic eye disease. With background retinopathy, your retina may contain some leaky or blocked capillaries, or a combination of the two. There may be tiny swellings in some of the capillaries, called microaneurysms. In most cases, background retinopathy does not present an immediate threat to your vision. However, if swelling or leakage occur near the macula, the macula may become inflamed. "Macular edema", as this is called, can lead to moderate or severe vision loss. You may need further testing or more frequent visits to your eye doctor to assess the progress of your retinopathy.

Preproliferative Retinopathy is the second stage in the progression of diabetic eye disease. When blood vessels are failing to deliver enough oxygen to parts of the retina, particularly the macula, white patches of oxygen-starved retina appear. These are called "cotton wool spots" because of their cottony appearance. Any time a part of the retina is deprived of oxygen, it sends out warning signals that stimulate the growth of new blood vessels. These new blood vessels will tend to grow in an uncontrolled manner (they "proliferate" the area).

Proliferative Retinopathy is the most severe and vision-threatening form of diabetic eye disease. When new blood vessels grow in the retina, they tend to grow in bunches. These bunches of blood vessels may cover up areas of the retina, preventing light from reaching through. This is sort of like putting your finger in front of the camera lens when taking a picture. The result will be major blind spots. If the new vessels grow over the macula, complete blindness can result.

To make matters worse, the new blood vessels tend to be weak and are susceptible to rupturing and leaking blood into the center of the eye (the "vitreous fluid"). This can cause everything you see to have a cloudy or red appearance.

Finally, damaged blood vessels may form scar tissue that attaches the retina to the fluid-filled sac in the center of the eye. As the scar tissue shrinks, the retina may be pulled away from the back portion of the eye. A "retinal detachment", as this is called, can severely reduce vision.

Preventing, Detecting and Treating Retinopathy

With all the problems diabetes can cause, it should be a relief to know that 50-90% of vision loss experienced by people with diabetes can be prevented. Good control of blood sugar is a big key to preventing diabetic eye problems. In the DCCT study, researchers found that tight control of blood sugar levels not only reduces the incidence of retinopathy by 50-70%, but also slows the progression of retinopathy in those who already have it. Keeping blood pressure under control and avoiding smoking and alcohol can also help prevent and slow the progression of eye disease.

Good control of diabetes can certainly lower your risk of eye problems, but it cannot guarantee good vision. Regular eye examinations are a must.

Unfortunately, most people with diabetes do not receive adequate eye care. Once retinopathy develops, it can proceed quickly. Vision loss or blindness can occur if eye disease is not treated in a timely manner. You can have significant damage to your retina before noticing any change in your vision. In most cases, the loss of vision is gradual and may not be noticed.

OPHTHALMOLOGIST

A medical doctor specializing in diagnosing and treating diseases of the eye. Unlike opticians (who specialize in correcting vision) and optometrists, ophthalmologists are skilled at screening for and treating diabetic eye disease.

As mentioned earlier, everyone with diabetes should see their eye doctor for a complete exam at least once a year. People with Type-II diabetes should begin seeing an ophthalmologist as soon as they are diagnosed; those with Type-I diabetes can begin five years after diagnosis. Women who have diabetes should have their eyes checked before becoming pregnant and regularly during the course of pregnancy.

During your eye exam, the doctor should dilate your eyes and use a special magnifying device and bright light to carefully examine the blood vessels in your retina. A casual look in your eyes during a routine visit to your doctor's office is not sufficient.

You should also see your ophthalmologist as soon as possible if you experience any of the following symptoms:

- Any abrupt change of vision in one eye

- Blurred vision that does not go away in a day

- Sudden loss of vision

- Black spots or floaters

- Cobwebs

- Flashing lights

- Eye pain

- "Pink Eye"

Through early detection, LASER TREATMENT can be used to clear up areas of the retina that are obscured by retinopathy. The laser focuses on parts of the retina that are not receiving adequate blood flow, and keeps them from signaling the growth of new blood vessels. When retinopathy is detected and treated early, laser treatment can prevent vision loss in a majority of cases.

If you value your vision (and you should), make it your responsibility to make an appointment with an ophthalmologist. Don't wait for your doctor to remind you. By then, it could be too late.

This, that and the other

Retinopathy is just one of many eye conditions related to diabetes. People with diabetes are at an increased risk for glaucoma, a problem with fluid movement within the eye. If not treated quickly, glaucoma can cause a painful increase in pressure within the eye. This pressure causes damage to the optic nerve (the nerve that transmits signals from the eye to the brain) and can lead to blindness.

Cataracts, which are clouded areas in the lens of the eye, occur at an earlier age and tend to be more severe in people with diabetes. High blood sugar also changes the shape of the lens of the eye, which can cause blurred vision or nearsightedness (difficulty seeing things at a distance). Try not to be fitted for eyeglasses or contact lenses until your blood sugar levels are under control and stable.

Key point:

Diabetic eye disease is serious but preventable. Keep your blood sugar under the best control possible, and have your eyes examined every year.

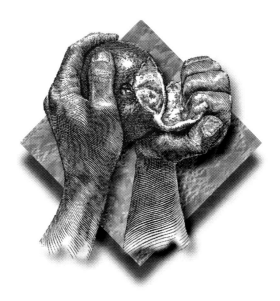

Chapter 28: Diabetes and Nerve Disease

There is little doubt that living with diabetes takes faith, confidence, persistence, and a take-charge attitude. Isn't it ironic that the same disease that requires a lot of nerve also can do extensive damage to the nerves?

"Neuropathy" means damage to the nerves. More than 10% of all people with diabetes suffer from neuropathy, with symptoms ranging from numbness in the feet to an inability to get an erection. Since the nerves are involved in so many bodily functions, the effects of neuropathy can be quite far-reaching.

Neuropathy is probably the most frustrating of the diabetic complications because it is so difficult to treat. Unlike retinopathy (eye disease), nephropathy (kidney disease) and heart disease, little can be done about neuropathy other than trying to lessen the symptoms and keep it from leading to more serious problems. However, in recent years, a great deal of progress has been made towards understanding why neuropathy develops and what can be done to prevent and/or treat it.

How nerves become damaged

Nerves are responsible for carrying signals between the brain (or spinal cord) and various parts of the body. Some nerves go from the body to the brain; they carry signals related to sight, sound, smell, taste and touch. Other nerves go from the brain to different parts of the body. They help coordinate our movements, speech, digestion, breathing, and countless other bodily functions.

Nerves carry signals by way of tiny electrical impulses. The nerves are like living electrical wires running all over the body. As long as the wires stay connected and are working properly, the nervous systems runs like clockwork. However, if the wires become damaged, they might "short circuit" - that is, they might fire continuously (not shut off) or not at all.

What is it about diabetes that causes damage to the nervous system? At present, we don't know the exact answer. But research has uncovered some important facts that link hyperglycemia (high blood sugar) to nerve damage:

1. Unlike the other parts of the body, nerve cells do not require insulin to get sugar inside. When the blood sugar level is high, a great deal of sugar enters the nerve cell. High levels of sugar in the cells trigger a chemical reaction that starts to corrode the outer part of the nerve fiber, sort of like stripping the rubber coating off an electrical cord. Without this coating, the nerve has a difficult time transmitting signals properly.

2. Remember, nerve is living tissue. It requires oxygen and nutrients to stay alive. We already know that diabetes can impair the circulation by damaging tiny blood vessels. Without adequate blood supply, some nerve fibers may die.

3. All animals have the ability to repair and renew damaged nerve fibers. In people with diabetes, nerve regeneration is abnormally slow. This may be due to low levels of Insulin-like Growth Factors (IGFs), which are natural substances that protect and spur the growth of nerves.

One thing we know for sure is that high blood sugar levels contribute to nerve damage. In the DCCT (Diabetes Control and Complications Trial), people who controlled their blood sugar carefully had 50-70% fewer nerve problems than people whose control was poor. In addition, people who already had neuropathy at the beginning of the study were able to slow, and in many cases reverse, the progression of nerve disease by taking better care of their diabetes.

The many forms of neuropathy

Different types of nerve damage result in different forms of neuropathy.

SENSORY NEUROPATHY

Sensory nerves (from skin to brain) carry sensations of pain, touch and pressure. When these nerves become damaged, it is possible to become overly sensitive to touch (pain may be constant) or insensitive to pain. This can happen as early as five years after diabetes is diagnosed, especially if blood sugar control is poor. Sensory neuropathy is the most common diabetic complication. It occurs with similar frequency in Type-I and Type-II diabetes, and its occurrence seems to parallel the duration and severity of high blood sugar.

Symptoms of sensory neuropathy include:

- "pins and needles" in the feet, legs or hands. Painful sensations may decrease over time as the nerves die off.
- numbness in the feet, legs or hands
- feeling as though you are walking on wool or cotton
- leg pain while lying in bed
- chronic foot or leg pain
- hypersensitivity to touch (clothing or bed sheets may be painfully irritating)

Sensory neuropathy is dangerous because it can eliminate one of the body's main sources of protection: PAIN. Pain tells us when we are hurting, and where the problem is. If you feel pain all or none of the time, you cannot rely on pain to tell you when something is wrong. You could burn yourself, cut your skin, twist an ankle, or develop a serious callus or blister without ever knowing it. Many people with diabetes lose their feet and legs because minor injuries go undetected and result in major infections that are difficult to treat. For this reason, sensory neuropathy is responsible for most limb amputations in people with diabetes.

Sensory neuropathy can be detected by your doctor in a routine office visit. Your doctor can touch your feet and legs with filaments of various thicknesses to see which ones you can and cannot feel. It is a quick, painless and reliable test.

Once sensory neuropathy is detected, you must take extra care of your feet so that foot injuries are prevented and detected early. Blood sugar control should also be intensified in order to slow the progression of neuropathy. In severe cases, improvements in blood sugar control can alleviate many of the symptoms of painful sensory neuropathy. Lamb's wool padding on the feet and between toes can also relieve some of the painful symptoms. Over-the-counter pain relievers like Zostrix cream and relaxation exercises can also provide relief in some cases. Elavil, and Mexitil tablets (150 mg) are prescription items that may help control the pain.

MOTOR NEUROPATHY

Motor nerves carry signals from the brain to the muscles. In addition to telling our muscles when to contract (so that we can move), motor nerves also coordinate complex movements that require the use of several different muscles simultaneously.

If the motor nerves become damaged, our ability to make fine adjustments to muscles may be impaired. Most often, the motor nerves that coordinate the muscles within the feet are affected by neuropathy. When this happens, the way you normally walk (your gait) can change. Even subtle changes in gait can result in new pressure points on the feet, which may lead to the formation of an ulcer (sore). New pressure points must be treated or they can become badly infected. A trained podiatrist can develop special inserts (orthotics) for your shoes to redirect your pressure points. See Chapter 30 for more details.

Occasionally, motor neuropathy and sensory neuropathy occur together. When this happens, the legs can become weak and painful,

---

PRESSURE POINTS

Spots on the bottoms and sides of the feet where pressure is greatest when we stand up and walk. Our natural pressure points have extra padding to prevent the formation of sores (ulcers) which can become infected and lead to possible amputation.

---

making a simple walk in the park seem like torture. In some people, motor neuropathy can impair fine motor skills (dexterity, coordination, precision). A gifted artist or technician could lose their skills due to the damage caused by motor neuropathy.

AUTONOMIC NEUROPATHY

Autonomic nerves carry signals from the brain to our internal organs. They are like "cruise control" for our body - they control functions such as breathing, heart rate, digestion, sexual arousal, and perspiration so that we do not have to consciously think about them.

Autonomic neuropathy, as you might have guessed, involves damage to the nerves that control these functions. More than half of all people with sensory neuropathy will also have autonomic neuropathy. The effects of autonomic neuropathy can be far-reaching and, in some cases, life-threatening.

Below are some of the more common forms of autonomic neuropathy:

1. Gastroparesis: When the nerves controlling the stomach become damaged, the stomach may be slow to empty food into the small intestine. The food just sits in the stomach, causing a sense of bloating and nausea. Gastroparesis often causes vomiting after meals or dry heaves in the morning. What's more, gastroparesis makes blood sugar control even more difficult since food may not reach the blood stream in a consistent manner. If the stomach empties slowly one day, low blood sugar may occur right after meals and blood glucose may start to go up between meals. Fast emptying may result in high blood sugar after meals.

2. Cardiovascular Neuropathy: The nervous system plays a key role in keeping the heart rate and blood pressure under constant control. When we exercise, the blood vessels dilate, and the heart

rate speeds up. When we stand up after sitting or lying down, the blood vessels constrict to allow blood flowing up to the brain.

When the nerves controlling the heart and blood vessels are not doing their job, several problems can occur. During exercise, the heart rate does not speed up and you may become fatigued very quickly as muscles are deprived of oxygen. Of course, heart rate will not be a reliable indicator of exercise intensity. A self-rating of perceived exertion is a better approach for measuring your intensity when exercising. An extended warm-up and cool-down and steady exercise intensity can also help make exercise safe for those with cardiovascular neuropathy.

POSTURAL HYPOTENSION

A sudden drop in blood pressure when getting up from a sitting or lying position. The moment blood fails to reach the brain, dizziness or fainting usually occurs.

When standing up after sitting or lying down, the blood vessels in the legs may not constrict properly. This will lead to a sudden drop in blood pressure, and may cause you to become very dizzy and fall or pass out. Compression stockings may alleviate the problem. Cutting back on diuretics (water pills) and caffeine can also help.

In addition, the sensory nerves within the heart muscle may fail to transmit pain signals to the brain in the event of a heart attack. Silent MI (myocardial infarction), as this is called, is very dangerous because it may keep you from seeking proper medical attention. Annual electrocardiograms and exercise stress tests are recommended for some people with diabetes.

3. <u>Thermoregulation</u>: Nerves are also responsible for triggering perspiration (sweating). Perspiring is critical for maintaining body temperature. Too little sweating can cause body temperature to rise; too much sweating can cause it to fall. When the nerves controlling perspiration are damaged, the result can be too much or too little sweating. Neuropathy can also trigger sweating at inappropriate times; in response to food, for example. For those with impaired or excessive perspiration, temperature extremes (very hot/humid weather and very cold weather) should be avoided.

4. <u>Excretion</u>: The muscles that control bowel movements and urination (emptying of the bladder) are controlled by autonomic nerves. Damage to these nerves can result in leakage of stools from the rectum, diarrhea, constipation, or sluggish bowel movements. If the muscles of the bladder become weak, the bladder may leak or fail to empty entirely (resulting in bladder infections).

5. <u>Pupillary response</u>: When the nerves controlling the pupil (opening of the eye) become damaged, the eye may not adjust well to bright light and darkness. Night vision may be particularly poor.

6. <u>Impotency</u>: Nerves that control erection and lubrication of the vagina can be affected by neuropathy. Almost half of all diabetic men over age 50 suffer from impotency. Treatment options include mechanical pumps, injectible medications, and prosthetic implants. Women may resort to lubricating gells prior to intercourse.

Hope and promises...

Although current technology does not offer a "cure" for neuropathy, there are still plenty of measures that can be taken to alleviate the symptoms of neuropathy and prevent it from causing significant damage:

1. Control your blood sugar

2. Take care of your feet

3. Know the symptoms of neuropathy

4. Get tested regularly for neuropathy.

In addition, keep watching the news and reading your diabetes magazines for the latest research in treating neuropathy. Already, two medications have been found to be effective for preventing, treating and alleviating the symptoms of neuropathy. They are:

ALDOSE REDUCTASE INHIBITORS, which keep high blood sugar levels from doing damage to nerve fibers, and IGF-II, a growth factor that helps damaged nerves repair themselves. Both of these medications are in clinical trials and may be available in the next few years.

Key point:

Neuropathy is the most common complication of diabetes and
is a major factor contributing to foot and limb amputation.
Meticulous foot care is critical if you have diabetic neuropathy.

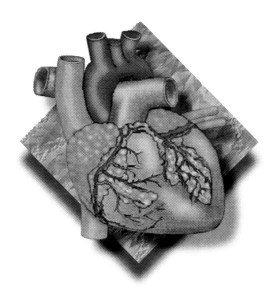

Chapter 29: The Heart of the Matter: Diabetes and Large Blood Vessel Disease

Ah... aging. A wonderful thing, isn't it? The stiff joints. The wrinkled skin. The appearance of a hair or two (or fifty) in the comb.

Oh, there is one other thing that happens as we age. It's called atherosclerosis, and it means that our large blood vessels (the ones that carry blood to major organs of the body) are becoming more narrow all the time. When blood vessels become narrow, organs like the heart, brain, skin and muscles may not be getting as much blood flow as they used to. If the blood flow becomes severely limited, it can result in a heart attack, stroke, leg pain, or poorly healing wounds.

MYOCARDIAL INFARCTION

Another name for a "heart attack". Insufficient oxygen will cause heart muscle to become weak and die. The heart loses its ability to pump blood if the heart muscle does not contract properly.

Heart disease is especially common among people with diabetes. More people with diabetes die from heart attacks than all other causes combined. When the heart muscle is deprived of oxygen, it starts to die. Typically, this will signal pain (angina), but it may not cause any pain if you have neuropathy. If a large enough portion of the heart is damaged, it will be difficult or impossible to recover.

CONGESTIVE HEART FAILURE

Due to impaired blood flow and/or weakened heart muscle, the heart may not be able to pump out all the blood it receives. As pressure builds up, breathing becomes impaired. Less oxygen is delivered to the heart muscle, resulting in further weakening and death of heart tissue.

When large blood vessels supplying oxygen to the brain become blocked, a portion of the brain can die. This is called a "stroke". If only a small portion of the brain is affected, the result may be a minor loss of motor skills or sensation. If a large portion is affected (massive stroke), significant physical and mental impairment or death can result.

Diabetes is also the leading cause of foot amputations. Typically, a minor injury such as a cut or sore is not detected due to neuropathy (insensitivity). As the injury becomes more severe, it may become infected. If the circulation to the foot is impaired, your body's defense systems (white blood cells, antibodies) will not be able to reach the infection to fight it. The infection becomes worse and worse until there is no other choice but to amputate the infected part of the body.

To better understand how this happens, imagine that you are the leader of a small army defending your hometown against a large, evil army. Your troops are being beaten, so you call for help. The cavalry rushes to your aid, but cannot find a road to the battle site. Before long, your troops become massacred and the evil army has gained enough momentum to ransack your hometown. Obviously, the ability to reach the battle site is key to fighting off attackers.

Why do blood vessels become narrow?

The exact reason why atherosclerosis occurs is still under intense investigation. We do know that there are several factors that can damage blood vessels and impair their ability to carry blood:

High blood pressure damages blood vessels by placing excessive strain on blood vessel walls and forcing the heart to work much harder than usual. Cracks in the blood vessel walls can lead to clotting and blockage of blood flow.

Smoking narrows blood vessels by causing the muscles surrounding arteries to constrict.

Chronic stress narrows blood vessels in a similar way.

Elevated cholesterol and triglycerides contribute to atherosclerosis by sticking to blood vessel walls and forming plaques which become progressively larger, narrowing the opening through which blood can flow.

Obesity damages blood vessels by raising triglycerides and blood pressure, and placing additional strain on the entire circulatory system.

Aging leads to progressive damage to blood vessels, as hardened arteries become less flexible and damage easily.

Low estrogen levels in post-menopausal women increase the risk for heart disease. Estrogen helps protect women against heart attack. For this reason, women with diabetes are twice as likely as men to have heart disease.

The bottom line is that blood vessels that once looked like this, with wide openings to carry lots of blood:

Now look like this, with a narrow opening or no opening at all:

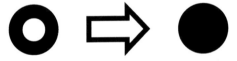

How does diabetes damage the circulation?

People with diabetes tend to develop narrowing of the arteries faster and more severely than people without diabetes. There are a number of reasons why this occurs, starting with high blood sugar.

Have you ever spilled something sweet? How does it feel after you wipe it up - sticky? Sugar has a way of sticking to LDLs in the blood-stream. The LDLs, in turn, stick to the walls of blood vessels, causing them to become progressively more narrow.

People with diabetes (especially Type-II diabetes) also tend to have high cholesterol, triglycerides and blood pressure. High blood pressure is three times more common in people with diabetes. Obesity is also present in 80% of people with Type-II diabetes. For these reasons, 50% of people with Type-II diabetes already have some narrowing of the coronary arteries (blood vessels supplying oxygen and nutrients to the heart) at the time they are diagnosed.

Another factor that leads to narrowing of the arteries is blood clotting. Clotting is a natural response to injury. Platelets (clotting cells in the blood) and special proteins clump together to fill cracks and holes to prevent blood loss. In people with diabetes, this clotting occurs more easily. Minor damage within blood vessel walls (caused by high blood pressure, obesity, etc.) leads to excessive clotting inside the blood vessel. This, in turn, contributes to hardening and thickening of the arteries.

(Too) Late diagnosis

Because of the increased risk of heart disease, people with diabetes should be aware of the early symptoms of heart trouble.

Typical symptoms of heart disease include chest pain (angina): tightness in the chest, pain in the left arm, shoulder or neck; numbness in the jaw; a sense of "pressure" in the chest; sharp pain in the stomach; or shortness of breath with mild exertion such as walking or taking a flight of stairs.

Too often, people ignore these symptoms or simply attribute them to a muscle cramp or indigestion. Any unusual pain should be checked by your doctor. Don't wait until you have a massive heart attack. Mild narrowing or blockages of coronary arteries can often be diagnosed and treated without surgery if caught early.

Your chances of surviving a heart attack are greatest when the blockage in an artery is dissolved within six hours. Unfortunately, many people with diabetes also have neuropathy. If the nerves leading from the heart are damaged, you may not feel the pain that usually occurs when the heart muscle is deprived of oxygen. Without a sense of pain to tell you when a heart attack has occurred, you may not receive treatment in time.

In people with diabetes, silent (painless) ischemia (Ischemia: Lack of oxygen) occurs four times more often than painful ischemia. The only way to find out if your heart is receiving adequate blood flow is through a routine electrocardiogram or exercise stress test.

Blood flow to the legs and feet can also be assessed before serious problems set in. If you experience pain in your legs or feet when walking, and the pain fades away when resting, you may have impaired circulation in your legs. Your doctor can check the pulses in your ankles to see if blood flow is sufficient.

Here comes the cavalry!

Just because diabetes puts you at a high risk for circulatory problems, don't get the feeling that there is nothing you can do about it. In fact, by doing the right things and taking good care of yourself, you could and should be able to prevent large blood vessel disease.

1. <u>Blood sugar control</u>: Keep your HbA1c as low as possible. An HbA1c less than 8% without a lot of low blood sugars is ideal. Look to keep your pre-meal blood sugars in the 90-120 range, and your post-meal blood sugars under 180.

2. <u>Healthy diet</u>: Eating plenty of fresh fruits, vegetables and fiber, and cutting down on fat (especially saturated fat) will lower your risk for atherosclerosis. When including fat in your diet, try to use

mono-unsaturated fat (the kind found in olive oil, canola oil, nuts and fish).

3. Exercise: 30 minutes or more of moderate cardiovascular exercise each day helps to lower cholesterol, triglycerides, blood sugar, blood pressure, body fat and clotting factors in the blood. Exercise also stimulates the growth of collateral circulation - new blood vessels that supply oxygen in case old blood vessels become blocked.

4. Blood pressure control: Keeping blood pressure under 140/90 alleviates strain on the heart and minimizes damage to the walls of blood vessels. Ace inhibitors and calcium channel blockers are the preferred medications for blood pressure control in people with diabetes.

5. Reduce cholesterol and triglycerides: Have your cholesterol and triglycerides checked annually. Keep them under 200 (and as low as possible) to prevent atherosclerosis.

6. Antioxidants: Antioxidants are chemicals that prevent substances in the blood from sticking to the walls of blood vessels. This, in turn, slows down and prevents hardening of the arteries. Vitamin E is one of the best antioxidants when used in small doses (400-800 units). Other antioxidants include beta carotene (found in carrots), selenium, zinc, garlic, onion, and ginseng.

7. Estrogen supplements: Before menopause, women have a low incidence of heart disease because of the protection offered by the hormone estrogen. Estrogen acts as an antioxidant. It also dilates (opens up) blood vessels, and increases HDLs (good cholesterol). After menopause, women stop making their own estrogen, and the risk of heart attack increases several fold. Therefore, most women (especially those with diabetes) are encouraged to take estrogen supplements after menopause in order to prevent heart attack.

8. <u>No smoking</u>: Smoking not only causes immediate and severe constriction of the blood vessels. It also impairs the blood's ability to transport oxygen, increases the level of LDL (bad cholesterol) in the blood, and reduces the effects of estrogen and other antioxidants.

These factors make smoking and diabetes the worst combination for heart attacks and other circulatory problems.

9. <u>Aspirin</u>: An aspirin a day (enteric-coated to prevent stomach upset) has been shown to reduce the risk of heart attack and repeat heart attack.

The bottom line

Large blood vessel disease is a serious progressive illness. Everyone has it to some degree, and it gets worse over time. Its effects are devastating - heart attack, stroke, limb amputation, and sudden death. And like it or not, simply having diabetes puts you at a much greater risk for circulatory problems.

To fight back, you must take a pro-active approach. That means reducing your risk factors before serious problems set in. Your lifestyle is the best place to start. Eat right, exercise regularly, and do your best to minimize stress. Have your circulation checked at least once a year by your doctor, and you should be able to head off heart disease and other circulatory problems at the pass.

Key point:

Heart disease is the number one killer of people with diabetes. Living healthy and keeping your blood pressure, cholesterol and weight under control are the first steps to preventing circulatory complications.

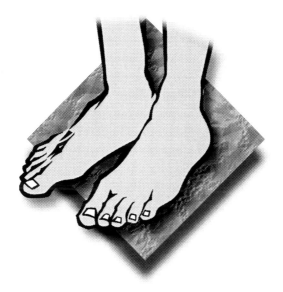

Chapter 30: Diabetes and Foot Infections

Early this morning, Joan called the office. Joan is a pleasant woman, but this morning she sounded out of sorts.

"I don't feel well," she said. "I think there's something wrong with my foot. It looks all swollen. Is there anything I can take for it?"

"Take a cab and come in right away," I told her.

She limped into the office with her foot wrapped in an Ace bandage from the corner drug store. She unwrapped the bandage halfway, and it didn't look good. She had an ulcer on the bottom of her foot that was so badly infected that we had to rush her to the hospital.

That was two hours ago. By this time tomorrow, Joan will no longer have a right foot.

As health care professionals, we are prepared to deal with all sorts of hardships and suffering that our patients endure. Still, it is difficult to keep from becoming emotional when something like this happens to a patient. Emotions can range from deep sadness to serious anger. What right does diabetes have to take this woman's foot? And why was something not done about it sooner?

The threat of foot ulcers, infections and amputations are a fact of life for people with diabetes. Each year, more than 50,000 people with diabetes have a toe, foot or entire limb amputated. THESE PROBLEMS MUST STOP. Yes, diabetes increases the risk for foot problems. But that does not excuse the fact that people with diabetes and their doctors neglect to take adequate care of the foot. Virtually every amputation can be prevented through proper hygiene, foot care, screening and treatment.

A healthy pair of feet is important. Your feet allow you to enjoy a healthy game of tennis, a walk in the park with someone you love, and a special dance at your granddaughter's wedding. If you are interested in keeping your feet healthy for a lifetime, read this chapter twice - once for each foot.

Why does diabetes lead to foot problems?

Understanding the problems that can affect your feet is the first step toward protecting them. First of all, we know that most people with diabetes lose at least some of the sensation in their legs and feet due to neuropathy (see chapter 28). Without adequate sensation, an injury can occur and you would never know it. For example, neuropathy may keep you from noticing:

- ill-fitting shoes
- a foreign object in your shoe
- a mild burn from walking on hot sand or pavement
- sunburn
- water that is too hot
- a cut or scrape
- blisters and calluses
- ingrown toenails
- dry, cracked skin

Without noticing and treating these types of problems, the damage can become quite severe. Compounding the problem is the fact that many people with diabetes have <u>peripheral vascular disease</u>, or poor circulation in the legs and feet (see chapter 29). When blood flow to an injury is limited, there may not be enough oxygen, nutrients and white blood cells (antibodies) to repair the area and fight infection. High blood sugar also decreases the ability of white blood cells to fight infection and destroy bacteria.

Infection can occur within the skin, the soft tissue below the skin, and even in the bones. People with diabetes are particularly prone to develop infections in the bones of the feet (osteomyelitis). <u>Infection</u> is caused by bacteria getting into the injured area (usually when there is a break in the skin) and spreading. Infection causes blood flow to be cut off even further. If infection is not treated quickly and appropriately, the tissue in the infected area will begin to die. This is called "gangrene". The dead tissue becomes a breeding ground for additional bacteria. Removal of the dead tissue is necessary to prevent the infection from spreading further. Gangrene may require amputating (cutting off) a toe, foot, or entire leg depending on the severity of the infection.

The diabetic foot ulcer: a problem waiting to happen.

A foot ulcer is a nasty sore caused by an injury that is made worse by repeated pressure on the area. The most common foot ulcers occur on the bottom of the foot. These are called plantar ulcers. They usually occur on the ball of the foot, just below the big toe, but they can occur in other places as well. Foot deformities such as claw toes or hammer toes can lead to ulcerations at the tips or tops of the toes.

Most often, a callus (thickening of the skin) forms and becomes irritated by continued pressure from walking or standing. As a result, the center of the callus becomes decayed, leaving the skin open to infection-causing bacteria. If not treated soon, the bacterial infection can spread, resulting in gangrene.

Treatment of diabetic food ulcers

An important factor in the development of a foot ulcer is increased pressure on a particular area of the foot. Careful trimming of the callus by a podiatrist can reduce the pressure by 30%. Wearing shoes, especially athletic or running shoes, can also decrease callus build-up. Walking barefoot tends to place the most pressure on a callus.

If an ulcer develops, you will need fast and aggressive treatment. An untreated or under-treated foot ulcer can result in serious infection which may require amputation. If you notice redness, swelling, pus, pain or callus buildup on your foot, get to your doctor as soon as possible. Treatment usually involves trimming away the callus and application of antibiotics. X-rays and bone scans are also in order, as bone can easily become infected.

The most important treatment for a foot ulcer is something you do yourself: STAY OFF THE FOOT ENTIRELY until your doctor says you can place pressure on it again. There are a variety of devices and techniques that will help you to get around without placing any pressure on your infected foot. Discuss them with your doctor.

When ulcers develop on the toes, special shoes are often required. The toe box must be large enough to avoid placing pressure on the ulcers, and a special insole is used to protect the bottom of the toes from ulceration. Putting an insole into an ordinary shoe may cause the tops of the toes to press against the shoe, resulting in further ulceration. An extra deep shoe is essential.

Therapeutic (molded) shoes are an effective way to prevent further ulceration. Studies have shown that people who wear therapeutic shoes after being treated for a foot ulcer only have a 20% chance of developing another ulcer. Those who do not wear therapeutic shoes have an 80% chance of recurrence.

Preventive measures: what you must do.

Sure, we have insurance companies with their managed care programs and preferred provider networks. We have doctors specializing in everything from foot fungus to bone scans. We have state-of-the-art technology, medications and surgical techniques. And we have bioengineering so advanced that we can re-build and repair just about every part of the body.

Even with all that, 50,000 Americans still need to have their toes, feet and limbs amputated each year. Which brings us to one crucial point: YOU, AND NOBODY BUT YOU, IS RESPONSIBLE FOR TAKING CARE OF YOUR FEET. Not your spouse, not your doctor, and certainly not your insurance company.

There is no reason that anybody with diabetes should lose a foot if they take good care of themselves. That means:

- Having your feet examined by a podiatrist at least once a year, even if you don't think there are any problems.

- Wearing shoes that fit properly. Try on new shoes at the end of the day when your foot has expanded. Do not buy shoes that are uncomfortable and expect them to "stretch".

- Inspecting your feet daily. Simply look at the tops and bottoms of your feet and between your toes for signs of cuts, scrapes, cracks, calluses, redness and swelling. Use a mirror if you have trouble seeing the bottoms of your feet, or have a family member check for you.

- Checking your shoes for foreign objects before putting them on.

- Avoiding burns. Use lukewarm water for bathing (test water temperature with your elbow), and do not walk barefoot on hot sand, pavement, or pool decks. Do not use hot water bottles, heating pads, hot compresses or heating lamps near your feet. Use a powerful sunscreen on the feet, legs and ankles to prevent sunburn.

- Keeping the skin moist. Dry skin is susceptible to cracking and allows bacteria to enter the body easily. Apply a moisturizer to your feet (except between the toes) after bathing/showering.

- Wearing thick cotton socks. Socks help absorb shock and perspiration, and keep the skin from rubbing against the insides of shoes.

- Wearing shoes whenever possible. Wear sneakers, sandals or slippers outdoors and indoors. Wear aqua-socks in and around water.

- Not soaking your feet. Soaking dries out the skin, making it easy for bacteria to penetrate. Soaking with cleansing agents and antibiotics will only treat bacteria on the skin surface and may cause tissue damage.

- NEVER PERFORMING HOME SURGERY ON YOUR FEET! Seek a foot care specialist (a podiatrist) for all foot treatments - major and minor.

- Staying away from over-the-counter medications to treat corns, calluses or problem toe nails. Many of these products contain acid that can cause permanent tissue damage. Only use medications prescribed by your doctor.

- Trimming nails properly. Trim toenails straight across and file the edges with an emery board. Never stick anything sharp under your toenails! If you have trouble trimming your own toenails, have a podiatrist do it for you.

- Keeping your blood sugar under control. Remember, high blood sugar can hurt your nerves and impair your circulation, and it makes infection more difficult to treat.

- Avoiding actions that impair the circulation, such as smoking, sitting with legs crossed, and wearing elastic garters.

Preventive measures: what your doctor must do.

Remember, your doctor is a paid consultant whose job is to protect and preserve your good health. Although ultimate responsibility for your foot care rests squarely on your shoulders, you should expect nothing less than the following from your doctor:

- A complete foot inspection (tops, bottoms, and between the toes) at every visit. Remove your shoes and socks every time you go into the exam room as a reminder.

- A close examination of the circulation in your feet (temperature and pulses) at least once a year.

- An annual test for sensory neuropathy by touching wire filaments to your feet.

- Referral to the right specialists (podiatrist, vascular specialist, neurologist, radiologist, orthotic fitter) at the earliest signs of foot problems.

To learn more about foot care and what you can do to prevent foot problems, contact the Professional Diabetes Academy for a copy of "Feet First", available in booklet or video form (see Appendix B).

Key point:

Don't become an amputation statistic. By practicing sound foot care, you should be able to keep your feet healthy for a lifetime.

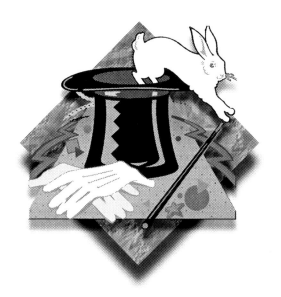

Appendix A:

Skim the Milk and Spare the Fat:
Basic Low-Fat Cooking Techniques

Substitutions

Skim away fat and calories from all sorts of recipes by trying some of these easy-to-use substitutions. Before long, your meals will be within healthful fat limits, and you won't have to sacrifice great taste!

For example, simply replacing whole milk (4% milkfat) with 2% milk will save 4 grams of fat and 36 calories per cup! Switching to skim milk will save another 4 grams of fat and 36 calories per cup.

Remember to limit your fat intake to no more than 30% of your total calorie intake.

If your daily calorie intake is...	Limit your daily fat intake to ...
1000 calories	33 grams
1200 calories	40 grams
1500 calories	50 grams
1800 calories	60 grams
2000 calories	67 grams
2500 calories	83 grams

The Evaporation Sensation

For a rich, creamy sauce or soup that is low in fat and calories, use evaporated skim milk instead of cream. Evaporated skim milk has a creamy flavor and is richer in texture than regular milk.

Abracadabra! Make more than 20 grams of fat and 180 calories disappear in every 1/4 cup served!

Sour on Sour Cream

Use non-fat or low-fat plain (or vanilla) yogurt in place of sour cream. Yogurt works great in stroganoff recipes, and even in ambrosia salad. In sauces, add 2 tablespoons of flour to each cup of yogurt so the sauce will thicken properly. In hot dishes, stir the yogurt just before serving, since high temperatures can cause yogurt to curdle. Alternatively, try light (reduced calorie, reduced fat) sour cream, or substitute part-skim ricotta cheese or low-fat cottage cheese blended with buttermilk. Be sure to compare labels to see if the substitute is really lower in fat and calories.

Hocus Pocus! Make up to 25 grams of fat and 200 calories disappear in every 1/4 cup!

An Applesauce A Day...

Many baked products call for high-fat oil, margarine or butter. Next time, try using applesauce instead. This substitution works well in muffins, quick breads, cake mixes, and cakes made from scratch. Applesauce is rich in a natural substance called "pectin" which helps baked goods come out moist and delicious.

Alacazam! Make 25 grams of fat and 200 calories disappear per 1/4 cup of butter which you replace with applesauce!

Apples & Buttermilk

In recipes where oil is the only liquid ingredient, use a combination of half applesauce and half low-fat buttermilk instead. Low-fat buttermilk is a good choice because it has more body than other liquids such as skim milk, fruit juice and water.

Shazam! Make 15 grams of fat and 75 calories disappear per 1/4 cup!

Prunes-A-Plenty

Pureed prunes or "baby food" prunes are an ideal fat replacer in chocolate baked goodies such as cakes and brownies. Prunes add a naturally sweet flavor and chewy texture to baked items. To puree prunes, place 2/3 cup (4 ounces) of pitted prunes and 3 tablespoons of hot water in a blender and blend until smooth.

Abracadabra! Make 75 grams of fat and almost 500 calories disappear per 2/3 cup!

Marshmallow Mania

Traditional frosting is extremely high in fat and calories, and tends to be very heavy. If you want to add fluff to your frosting, replace the margarine or butter with marshmallow creme. Marshmallow adds creaminess without contributing any fat.

Hocus Pocus! Make 100 calories disappear per slice of cake!

Better Than Butter

If a recipe calls for "solid" fat like butter, margarine or shortening, try replacing it with a reduced-calorie liquid margarine. These products are made lighter by having water whipped into them. It is generally best to use these products in foods that won't be cooked. In some recipes, such as cookies, the water from the margarine will change the texture of the final product.

Alacazam! Make 30 grams of fat and almost 300 calories disappear per 1/4 cup!

No Excuse. Just Add Juice.

For a nonfat salad dressing or marinade, use fruit juice. White grape, apple, orange, and pineapple juices are all refreshing, light alternatives to oil-based dressings. For a less fruity taste, combine the juice with defatted chicken broth.

Shazam! Make 50 to 100 calories disappear per 2 tablespoons!

Yank Them Yolks

When a recipe calls for a whole egg, use two egg whites instead. To de-yolk eggs, pour the egg into a glass and spoon out the entire yolk in one piece, if possible. Egg whites offer excellent texture and consistency to recipes.

Abracadabra! With each yolk you eliminate, you will make 5 grams of fat (45 calories) and a whopping 225 milligrams of cholesterol disappear!

Shimmy, Shimmy, Cocoa Powder

For great chocolate flavor without the fat, use cocoa powder. For each ounce of unsweetened chocolate, substitute 3 tablespoons of unsweetened cocoa powder. Adding 1/2 to 1 teaspoon of instant coffee granules further enhances the texture and chocolate flavor.

Alacazam! Watch 20 grams of fat and over 150 calories disappear!

Can The Soup

Remember those fattening cream soups you used to buy for use in casseroles? Can 'em! Making your own low-fat cream soup is a snap. In a small saucepan, use a wire whisk to stir together 1 cup of evaporated milk, 1 tablespoon cornstarch, and 1 teaspoon of low-sodium bouillon granules. Heat and stir until thickened and bubbly, then continue cooking and stirring for 1 minute more.

Hocus Pocus! Make 120 calories magically disappear!

Smile and say, "Low Fat Cheese!"

Instead of using whole-milk ricotta cheese, use part-skim ricotta or 1% fat cottage cheese. Regular cream cheese can be replaced with Neufchatel or reduced fat cream cheese. You can also combine these with plain nonfat yogurt, part-skim ricotta or low-fat cottage cheese. Additionally, mozzarella lovers can replace whole-milk mozzarella with a part-skim version.

Abracadabra! These cheesy substitutions eliminate plenty of fat and calories, and you will hardly taste the difference!

Mayo Makeover

Instead of high-fat mayonnaise, use plain yogurt, reduced-calorie mayonnaise, or low-fat cottage cheese. For a real treat, make your own "mock mayonnaise" by mixing 1/2 cup reduced calorie, low-fat mayonnaise with 1/2 cup low-fat plain yogurt.

Alacazam! Make 4 grams of fat and 34 calories disappear per tablespoon!

Now You're Cookin'!

To replace some or all of the fat (oil) when stir-frying, simmering or sautéing, use low-sodium broth, wine, beer or fruit juice instead.

Shazam! Make 20 to 50 calories disappear per serving!

Dressing for Success

Instead of high-fat dressings, use this almost-fat-free recipe. It also makes a great dip!

- 1 Small envelope (1 oz.) ranch dressing powder (reduced calorie)
- 1 1/2 cups nonfat milk
- 1/2 cup nonfat plain yogurt
- 1 tablespoon reduced-fat, reduced-calorie mayonnaise

Blend the milk, yogurt, mayo and powder together well. Refrigerate; stays good for about five days. Makes 2 cups.

Flavoring Without Fat

Flavor is the main feature that makes foods appealing. Often, fat is responsible for giving food much of its flavor. When you want to get rid of the fat but keep the flavor, try some of these expert flavoring tips:

Extracts

Keep extracts on hand to use as a convenient, fat-free flavoring agent. Some of the more popular ones include almond, mint, lemon, rum, vanilla, coconut, butter, orange, and liquid smoke. Liquid flavorings such as low-sodium soy sauce and flavored vinegars can also do the trick.

Veggies

Vegetables and vegetable flavorings such as ginger root, onion, celery, garlic shallot and horseradish can bring a variety of dishes to life without using fattening sauces and gravies.

Fruits

Certain fruits make excellent dressings and seasonings. Try using lemon, lemon peel, oranges, orange peel, limes, grapefruit, or fruit purees (berries, melons, peaches, prunes or dried apricots).

Herbs & Spices

Experimenting with different herbs and spices in various recipes isn't just healthy... it's fun! Start your herb collection with some proven favorites: basil, dill, tarragon, oregano, cumin, coriander, ground pepper, thyme, sage, and garlic powder.

Sweeteners

Flavored sweeteners such as molasses, brown sugar, maple syrup and concentrated fruit juices are a great way to add taste without adding fat.

Liqueurs

Give everyday dishes a little extra kick with orange or coffee-flavored liqueurs, amaretto, vermouth, sherry, wine, beer, or creme de menthe.

Fat Replacement Reminders

Ever receive one of those "You May Already Be a Winner" letters from Ed McMahon? Sure, the entry is free, but you still have to read through tons of product literature and spend half an hour filling out forms. Just goes to remind us that there is no such thing as a free lunch.

When you take the fat out of a recipe, you can't expect the food to taste exactly the same. Often, it is necessary to add a liquid ingredient (preferably with little or no fat) to make up for the volume and moistening power of the fat that was removed.

With the flavoring and substitution strategies given here, you are well on your way to lowering the fat content of your meals and still having food that looks and tastes darned close to the original.

Here are a few specific examples:

In muffins and nut breads, use only 2 tablespoons of oil, butter or margarine per 12-muffin recipe. To make up the remainder of the recipe, use reduced-calorie margarine or applesauce.

In homemade cakes or cookies, reduce the fat ingredient (usually butter) by about 50%. For the remainder, substitute something compatible with the flavor of the cookie or cake, such as nonfat sour cream, applesauce, pineapple juice, flavored yogurt, evaporated skim milk, or pureed baby fruits.

In biscuits, reduce the fat from 1/2 cup to 4 tablespoons per 2 cups of flour by substituting nonfat sour cream or light cream cheese to make up the difference.

In pie crust, reduce the fat to 3 tablespoons per cup of flour, and add 3 tablespoons of water.

In cheese sauce, eliminate butter and margarine altogether. Make a thickening paste by mixing flour with a little bit of skim milk, add the cheese, and whisk in more milk to get the consistency you want.

Eliminate the oil in tomato sauces. Instead, add herbs and spices to vary the flavor.

In marinades, the fat ingredient serves no important purpose. Use wine instead.

Appendix B: Resources

American Association of Diabetes Educators (AADE)
Providers of: Referral service for Certified Diabetes Educators
444 N. Michigan Ave.
Suite 1240
Chicago, IL 60611-3901
800-TEAM-UP-4

American Diabetes Association (ADA)
Publishers of: Diabetes Forecast magazine
1660 Duke St.
Alexandria, VA 22314
703-549-1500
800-232-3472

Atwater Carey, Ltd.
Makers of: Dia-Pak supply cases
5505 Central Ave.
Boulder, CO 80301
800-359-1646
303-444-9326

Bayer Corporation
Makers of: Glucometer Elite and Glucometer Encore blood glucose meters
511 Benedict Ave.
Tarrytown, NY 10591
800-348-8100

Becton-Dickinson (B-D) Consumer Products
Makers of: Syringes, Home Sharps Containers, Magni-Guide, B-D Pen, Disposable Syringes, Lancet Device, Ultra-Fine Lancets and B-D Glucose Tablets.
One Becton Drive
Franklin Lakes, NJ 07417-1883
800-237-4554

Boehringer Mannheim Corp.
Makers of: Accu-Chek Instant, Accu-Chek Easy, Accu-Chek III and Accu-Chek Advantage blood glucose meters; Softclix lancing device; and Accu-Chek PDM Pro data management software
9115 Hague Rd.
PO Box 50100
Indianapolis, IN 46250
800-845-7355

Can-Am Care Corporation
Makers of: Dex4 Glucose Tablets, Quick-Check generic blood glucose test strips, Monoject insulin syringes.
Cimetra Industrial Park
Box 98
Chazy, NY 12921
800-461-7448

Cascade Medical, Inc.
Makers of: Checkmate Plus blood
glucose meter
10180 Viking Dr.
Eden Prairie, MN 55344
800-525-6718
612-941-7345

Chronimed
Makers of: Quick Check One
generic test strips
13911 Ridgedale Drive
Suite 250
Minneapolis, MN 55305
800-444-5951
612-541-0239

Diabetic Insulcap, Inc.
Makers of: Insulcap
1606 Presidio Way
Roseville, CA 95661
916-781-3079

The Diabetic Traveler
Publishers of: The Diabetic Traveler
newsletter
P.O. Box 8223 RW
Stamford, CT 06905
203-327-5832

Disetronic Medical Systems, Inc.
Makers of: Disetronic Insulin
Pumps, Syringes and Infusion Sets
5201 East River Rd.
Suite 312
Minneapolis, MN 55421
800-280-7801
612-571-6878

EnviroTech of America, Inc.
Makers of: Sharps Containers
798 Hartwell Ave.
PO Box 239
East Syracuse, NY 13057
315-463-7178

Health-Mor Personal Care Corp.
Makers of: AdvantaJet and GentleJet
insulin injectors
185 E. North St.
Bradley, IL 60915
800-991-4464
815-932-5570

HealthWare
Makers of: Level data management
software
PO Box 5396
Buena Park, CA 90620
800-682-9375

Home Diagnostics, Inc.
Makers of: Diascan, Prestige and
Ultra blood glucose meters; and
Diascan Partner blood glucose meter
voice module
2300 NW 55th Court
Ft. Lauderdale, FL 33309
800-342-7226
954-677-9201

ICN Pharmaceuticals, Inc.
Makers of: Insta-Glucose gel
3300 Hyland Ave.
Costa Mesa, CA 92626
800-322-1515
714-545-0100

International Diabetic Athletes Ass.
Providers of: Networking and
support for sports and exercise
participation
1647 W. Bethany Home Rd.
Suite B
Phoenix, AZ 85015
800-898-IDAA
602-230-8155

Jordan Medical Enterprises
Makers of: Instaject, Count-A-Dose
202 Oaklawn Ave.
South Pasadena, CA 91030
800-541-1193
818-799-0317

Juvenile Diabetes Foundation (JDF)
Publishers of: Countdown magazine
432 Park Ave. South
New York, NY 10016
800-JDF-CURE
212-889-7575

Kings Publishing
Publishers of: Diabetes Interview
newspaper
3715 Balboa St.
San Francisco, CA 94121
415-387-4002

LifeScan, Inc.
Makers of: One Touch Basic, One
Touch Profile and Sure Step blood
glucose meters; and In Touch data
management software
1000 Gibraltar Drive
Milpitas, CA 95035
800-227-8862
408-263-9789

Lighthouse Consumer Products
Makers of: Touch -n- Talk III blood
glucose meter voice module
36-20 Northern Blvd.
Long Island City, NY 11101
800-829-0500

Medic Alert Foundation
Makers of: Medical identification
medallions and database
2323 Colorado Ave.
Turlock, CA 95382
800-432-5378

MediCool, Inc.
Makers of: Insulin Protector and
Protect All carrying cases
23761 Madison St.
Torrance, CA 90505
800-433-2469
310-375-4774

MediJect Corporation
Makers of: MediJector insulin
injector
1840 Berkshire Ln.
Minneapolis, MN 55441
800-328-3074
612-553-1102

MediLife, Inc.
Makers of: Balance PC data
management software
30 Monument Square
Concord, MA 01742
888-656-5656, x-2000

MediSense, Inc.
Makers of: ExacTech, MediSense 2
Card, MediSense 2 Pen and
Precision QID blood glucose meters;
and Precision Link data
management software
266 Second Ave.
Waltham, MA 02154
800-537-3575
617-895-6000

MedPort, Inc.
Makers of: MedPort supply cases
23 Acorn St.
Providence, RI 02903
800-299-5704
401-273-0630

MiniMed Technologies
Makers of: MiniMed Insulin Pumps,
Syringes, Infusion Sets, Books and
Accessories
12744 San Fernando Rd.
Sylmar, CA 91342
800-933-3322

Miles Inc. (Ames) Diagnostics Div.
Makers of: Ketostix
P.O. Box 70
Elkhart, IN 46515
800-348-8100

Novo Nordisk Pharmaceuticals, Inc.
Makers of: Novolin Insulin, Novolin
Prefilled Insulin Pens, Novo 1.5
Insulin Pen, Disposable Needles
Princeton, NJ 08540
800-727-6500

Palco Laboratories
Makers of: Inject-Ease injection aid,
Auto Lancet lancing device, and
InsulTote carrying case
8030 Soquel Ave.
Santa Cruz, CA 95062
800-346-4488
408-476-3151

Polymer Technology International
Makers of: First Choice generic test
strips
1871 NW Gilman Blvd.
Issaquah, WA 98027
800-877-2343

Professional Diabetes Academy
Publishers of: Feet First booklet and
video
777 East Park Dr.
PO Box 8820
Harrisburg, PA 17105
717-558-7750

R.A. Rapaport Publishing, Inc.
Publishers of: Diabetes Self-
Management magazine
150 W. 22nd St.
New York, NY 10011
800-234-0923
212-989-0200

Stat Medical Devices, Inc.
Makers of: Insul-Guide injection
aid, and Qwik-Let lancing device
1835 NE 146th St.
North Miami, FL 33181
(305) 945-0011

Superintendent of Documents
Publishers of: "The Medicare
Handbook"
Washington, DC 20402-9325
(202) 783-3238

Whittier Medical, Inc.
Makers of: Tru Hand
865 Turnpike St.
North Andover, MA 01845
800-645-1115
508-688-5002

INDEX

Suggested Readings

American Diabetes Association. "Self Monitoring of Blood Glucose." Consensus statement. Diabetes Care 17.1 (January 1994): 81-86.

Babione, Lois. "SMBG." Diabetes Spectrum 7.3 (1994): 198-199.

Bantle, John P. "Injection Site Rotation." Practical Diabetology 9.5 (1990): 1-4.

Barzilan, Nir. "Clinical Use of Metformin in the United States." Diabetes Spectrum 8.4 (1995): 194-197.

Beaser, Richard S. "Putting DCCT into Practice." Patient Care 29.3 (1995): 15-30.

Bell, David S. H. "Help for Brittle Diabetes." Diabetes Forecast 47.12 (1994): 36-40.

Chitwood, Marti. "Alcohol, Alcohol, Everywhere." Diabetes Forecast 46.11 (1992): 38-42.

Cryer, Philip E. et. al. "Hypoglycemia." Diabetes Care 17.7 (1994): 734-755.

Daly, Anne. "Carbohydrate Counting." Practical Diabetology 15.1 (1996): 19-23.

Davidson, Jaime A. et. al. "Non-Insulin Dependent Diabetes Mellitus in Hispanic-Americans." A round table discussion. Upjohn (1987): 3-22.

Fahey, Patrick J. et. al. "The Athlete with Type I Diabetes: Managing Insulin, Diet and Exercise." American Family Physician 53.5 (1996): 1611-17.

Farkas-Hirsch, Ruth. "Continuous Subcutaneous Insulin Infusion." Diabetes Spectrum 7.2 (1994): 80-84, 136-38.

Ferentz, Kevin S. "Recognizing and Treating Dysthymia in the Primary Care Patient." A Special Report: Depression in Primary Care December 1995: 13-20.

Goldstien, David. "The Test with a Memory." Diabetes Forecast. 47.5 (1994): 22-25.

Graham, Claudia. "Exercise in the Elderly Patient with Diabetes." Practical Diabetology 10.5 (1991): 8-11.

Guthrie, Richard. "Intensive Insulin Therapy for Insulin Dependent Diabetes." Internal Medicine 13.9 (1992): 35-44.

Hadden Dr. et. al. "Maturity Onset Diabetes Mellitus: Response to Intensive Dietary Management." Br Med. J. 3 (1975): 276-78.

Heaphy, Clifford John. "Facing Complications." Diabetes Forecast 46.5 (1993): 28-31.

Jaspan, Jonathan B. "Taking Control of Diabetes." Hospital Practice 30.10 (1995): 55-62.

Ko, Wilson. "Nonretinal Eye Problems in Diabetes." Practical Diabetology 9.5 (1990): 20-23.

Lebovitz, Harold E. "Management of Type II Diabetes Mellitus." American Family Physician. Monograph No. 1 (1995): 1-21.

Levandoski, Lucy A. et. al. "How to Get Tight Control - Safely." Diabetes Forecast 48.8 (1995): 24-27, 30-31.

Levin, Marvin E. "Preventing Amputation in the Patient with Diabetes." Diabetes Care 18.10 (1995): 1383-94.

Lorber, Daniel L. "Complications of Diabetes: Eye Disease." Practical Diabetology 12.4 (1993): 14-18.

McCarren, Marie. "The Mysterious Syndrome X." Diabetes Forecast 46.3 (1993): 42-45.

Morrow, Linda A. "Aging Well with Diabetes." Diabetes Forecast 46.3 (1993): 42-45.

Muir, Andrew et. al. "The Pathogenesis Prediction and Prevention of Insulin Dependent Diabetes Mellitus." Endocrinology and Metabolic Clinics of North America 21.2 (1992): 199-219.

Nolte, Martha S. "Insulin Therapy in Insulin Dependent (Type I) Diabetes." Endocrinology and Metabolic Clinic of North America 21.2 (1992): 281-305.

Orzeck, Eric A. "1500 Rules" (Personal Communication).
Piziak, Veronica K. "Attaining Maximum Benefit from Insulin Therapy." Contemporary Internal Medicine 7.2 (1995): 28-42.

Puczynski, Sandra. "Management of Nocturnal Hypoglycemia in IDDM." <u>Practical Diabetology</u> 13.3 (1994): 2-6.

Reasoner, Charles, "Diabetic Nephropathy: Pathogenetic Basis for Treatment." <u>Contemporary Internal Medicine</u> 6.10 (1994): 30-40.

Robbins, David C. "Acarbose a New Approach to Treating Type II Diabetes." <u>Practical Diabetology</u> 15.1 (1996): 2-8.

Robinson, Jennifer G. et. al. "Practical Management for Hyperlipidemia." <u>Contemporary Internal Medicine</u> 7.2 (1995): 15-27.

Sobel, Robert J. "Brittle Diabetes: Lessons for Optimizing Insulin Therapy." <u>Practical Diabetology</u> 13.1 (1994): 12-22.

Tilley, Belinda M. "Your Friendly Pharmacist." <u>Diabetes Forecast</u> 47.5 (1994): 48-50.

Victor, R. G. "Alcohol and Blood Pressure - A Drink a Day." <u>The New England Journal of Medicine</u> 332.26 (1995): 1782-83.

White, John R. "Ace Inhibitors and Their Role in Diabetes Mellitus." <u>Diabetes Spectrum</u> 6.3 (1993): 198-200.

White, Neil H. "The Risk of Hypoglycemia During Intensive Therapy of IDDM." <u>Diabetes Spectrum</u> 7.4 (1994): 232-33, 262-65.

Wing, R. R. et. al. "Long Term Effects of Modest Weight Loss in Type II Diabetes." <u>Archives of Internal Medicine</u> 147 (1987): 1749-53.

Zonszein, Joel. "Magnesium and Diabetes." <u>Practical Diabetology</u> 10.2 (1991): 1-5.

Zonszein, Joel, et. al. "Autonomic Neuropathy and Gastroparesis Diabeticorum." <u>Practical Diabetology</u> 10.5 (1991): 14-17.

About The Authors

Abdul Ghani, MD has been in private practice specializing in Diabetes and Internal Medicine for more than 20 years. Through his practice - The Midtown Clinic - located in Zephyrhills, Florida, he has successfully empowered thousands of individuals to take better control of their diabetes.

Dr. Ghani's passion for his work stems from a number of close friends and family members who were lost many years ago to the devastating complications of diabetes. Dr. Ghani believes that people have a right and an *obligation* to know how to take better care of themselves.

A native of Pakistan, Dr. Ghani graduated from King Edward Medical College in Lahore, Pakistan in 1969, and completed his internship at Catholic Medical Center of Brooklyn and Queens, New York in 1971. His residency in Internal Medicine and Fellowship in Endocrinology brought him to Cook County Hospital in Chicago from 1972 - 1975. Dr. Ghani currently serves on the staff of Columbia Dade City Hospital in Dade City, Florida, and East Pasco Medical Center in Zephyrhills, Florida.

Gary Scheiner, MS, CDE is a certified diabetes educator and exercise physiologist with a private practice in Merion, Pennsylvania. Having had Type-I diabetes since 1985, Gary uses his professional skills and personal experiences to teach people the "art and science of blood sugar balancing." A current insulin pump user, Gary is also a Certified Insulin Pump Trainer and Jet Injection Trainer.

Gary serves on the Board of Directors of the Juvenile Diabetes Foundation and American Diabetes Association, Philadelphia Chapters. He also plays an active role with the International Diabetic Athletes Assoc.

A frequent presenter at local and national meetings, Gary has written dozens of articles, both regionally and nationally, on diabetes, fitness and motivation. He earned a Bachelors degree in Psychology from Washington University in St. Louis, and a Masters degree in Exercise Physiology from Benedictine University.